Post Covid-19 Neurological Syndrome

Tissa Wijeratne • Sheila Crewther
Editors

Post Covid-19 Neurological Syndrome

A Pathway to SDG-3

Springer

Editors
Tissa Wijeratne
Department of Neurology and Stroke
La Trobe University
St. Albans, VIC, Australia

Sheila Crewther
Department of Neuroscience
La Trobe University
St. Albans, VIC, Australia

ISBN 978-3-032-14994-7 ISBN 978-3-032-14995-4 (eBook)
https://doi.org/10.1007/978-3-032-14995-4

This Springer imprint is published by the registered company Springer Nature Switzerland AG
The registered company address is: Gewerbestrasse 11, 6330 Cham, Switzerland

Foreword

It is with great pleasure that I write the foreword to this important volume on *Post-COVID Neurological Syndrome (PCNS)*, edited by Professors Tissa Wijeratne and Sheila Crewther. The COVID-19 pandemic has been the greatest public health challenge of our time, reshaping healthcare systems and leaving a legacy of uncertainty. Among the most complex legacies is the spectrum of neurological manifestations that persist well beyond the acute infection. These syndromes collectively described as PCNS have emerged as a pressing challenge for clinicians, researchers, and patients alike. Nevertheless, the pandemic has provided many learning opportunities to build a healthier tomorrow.

During the pandemic, the World Federation of Neurology (WFN) took a leading role in documenting and disseminating knowledge on the neurological complications of COVID-19. I had the privilege of coordinating the WFN's initiatives on COVID-19 and neurological manifestations, which highlighted both the enormous scale of the problem and the urgent need for systematic study. We quickly learned that the burden of PCNS extended across all regions and resource settings, with profound implications for patients' quality of life, healthcare delivery, and global brain health.

This book arrives at a crucial moment. It brings together cutting-edge insights from clinical practice, epidemiology, systems neuroscience, and rehabilitation, offering a comprehensive overview of the mechanisms, manifestations, and management strategies for PCNS. The editors and contributing authors have succeeded in bridging basic science and clinical application, while also highlighting the human and societal dimensions of this condition.

I commend Professors Wijeratne and Crewther for their leadership in assembling such an outstanding body of work. This volume will serve as both a practical resource for clinicians and a foundation for future research. Above all, it reminds us that the neurological consequences of COVID-19 must remain at the forefront of global health discourse long after the pandemic itself has receded.

Chandrasekhar Meshram

World Federation of Neurology
Convener, COVID-19 and Neurological
Manifestations Initiatives During the Pandemic
Director, Brain and Mind Institute
Nagpur India

President, AIIMS
Bibinagar, Hyderabad India

Preface

The COVID-19 pandemic has irrevocably transformed global health, not only by causing acute respiratory illness in millions but also by revealing a new and under-recognized frontier of post-viral disease. While the world mobilized to address the immediate crisis of SARS-CoV-2 infection, a second, quieter epidemic was unfolding in its wake: the prolonged and often disabling symptoms experienced by survivors long after the initial infection resolved. Among these, a condition now recognized as *Post-COVID Neurological Syndrome* (PCNS) has emerged as one of the most concerning and widespread sequelae of COVID-19.

PCNS refers to a constellation of persistent neurological and systemic symptoms that appear or persist after the acute phase of COVID-19. These include cognitive impairment, autonomic dysfunction, chronic fatigue, mood disturbances, sensory deficits, and neuropathic pain. In clinical practice, these symptoms often overlap and fluctuate, defying simple classification. Yet their impact on individuals and society is undeniable. Patients frequently describe their experiences as life-altering, with disruptions to memory, attention, and the ability to carry out basic daily tasks. The syndrome spares no age group, affecting both young adults and older individuals, and often appears even in those who had only mild or asymptomatic COVID-19 infections.

Our journey into understanding PCNS began early in the pandemic, when scattered reports of lingering symptoms began to emerge from various parts of the world. As a frontline neurologist and a molecular biologist, we both were among the first to systematically analyze these post-COVID presentations. In 2020, we proposed the term *Post-COVID Neurological Syndrome (PCNS)* to define this entity, advocating for a systems-based approach to its study, management, and policy recognition. What started as anecdotal observations rapidly evolved into a global health imperative, as it became clear that PCNS was not a rare complication, but a common and disabling outcome of SARS-CoV-2 infection.

Early epidemiological estimates have suggested that PCNS may affect between 5% and 50% of COVID-19 survivors. These figures vary depending on the population studied, the criteria used to define symptoms, and the duration of follow-up. Regardless of the exact prevalence, the scale of the pandemic means that tens of millions globally are likely to experience PCNS symptoms. This represents not only a major clinical challenge but also a social and economic crisis. Individuals with PCNS often face disruptions to work, education, and social engagement, while health systems struggle to meet the rising demand for neurological and rehabilitative services.

The syndrome's wide spectrum of symptoms can affect nearly every domain of functioning. Cognitive issues, often referred to as "brain fog," encompass problems with memory, attention, processing speed, and executive function. Autonomic disturbances manifest as orthostatic intolerance, palpitations, temperature dysregulation, and gastrointestinal irregularities. Sensory disturbances, such as anosmia and paresthesia, along with profound fatigue and mood changes, compound the burden. The persistent nature of these symptoms has led many patients to feel misunderstood or dismissed, emphasizing the need for healthcare providers to validate and address their concerns.

Scientific inquiry into PCNS has identified several plausible mechanisms. Neuroinflammation, often triggered by a dysregulated immune response, is a central factor. Elevated pro-inflammatory cytokines and evidence of blood-brain barrier dysfunction suggest that SARS-CoV-2 may incite a prolonged immune cascade that disrupts neural homeostasis. Mitochondrial dysfunction has also been implicated, potentially explaining the fatigue and cognitive slowing reported by many patients. In parallel, microvascular and endothelial damage—well documented in acute COVID-19—may impair cerebral perfusion and contribute to neurocognitive symptoms. The overlap of these mechanisms creates a complex, multifactorial syndrome that requires an equally multifaceted response.

Understanding who is most at risk of PCNS remains a critical gap. Current data suggest that women and older adults are more frequently affected, but younger, previously healthy individuals are by no means spared. Comorbidities such as asthma, autoimmune conditions, and preexisting mental health issues may increase susceptibility. Importantly, psychosocial factors—including stress, social isolation, and economic hardship—likely interact with biological processes to influence symptom persistence and severity.

In low- and middle-income countries (LMICs), the challenge is even more acute. Surveillance systems are often inadequate to track post-acute outcomes, and access to neurological care is limited. The burden of PCNS in these settings is likely underrecognized, underreported, and undertreated. The social determinants of health poverty, limited education, and fragile health infrastructure amplify the consequences of the syndrome. There is a pressing need for equity-driven research and investment to understand and address PCNS in LMIC contexts.

This book is a collaborative effort to address these challenges. It brings together experts in neurology, epidemiology, rehabilitation, public health, and health policy to explore the full scope of PCNS. Drawing on data from the Global Burden of Disease (GBD) 2022 study and frontline clinical observations, we examine the epidemiology, pathophysiology, health system impacts, and care models needed to respond to this crisis. The aim is not only to inform but to inspire: to catalyze coordinated action among researchers, clinicians, policymakers, and advocates.

As we move into the next phase of pandemic recovery, we must not lose sight of those still suffering. PCNS is a reminder that the health consequences of COVID-19 are not behind us. Rather, they continue to unfold in the lives of millions. It is our responsibility as a global health community to respond with urgency, compassion, and scientific rigor.

We dedicate this book to the patients who have endured PCNS with courage, to the clinicians who have listened and learned, and to the researchers and advocates who continue to shine light on this complex and evolving syndrome.

St. Albans, VIC, Australia

Tissa Wijeratne
Sheila Crewther

Introduction to Post COVID-19 Neurological Syndrome (PCNS): A Pathway to SDG-3

Introduction

In 2020, as the world grappled with the immediate threat of SARS-CoV-2, few could foresee the shadow it would cast in the years to come. While acute respiratory infection dominated early headlines, it soon became evident that the virus left lingering effects in a subset of individuals. These post-viral sequelae, often dismissed as nonspecific or psychosomatic, have since crystallized into a complex and disabling syndrome now widely recognized as Post COVID-19 Neurological Syndrome (PCNS).

As early as 2020, several members of this author group, including Wijeratne and Crewther, raised the alarm on emerging neurological patterns seen in patients post-COVID. From the onset, we were observing not just isolated cases of brain fog or fatigue but clusters of symptoms suggestive of systemic neuroimmune dysregulation. These cases were not confined to ICU survivors or elderly patients with comorbidities. Many were previously healthy individuals, including young adults and adolescents, who found themselves unable to return to work, school, or normal life months after recovering from the acute phase.

The need to define, name, and understand this condition led to the coining of PCNS, moving beyond vague terms like "long COVID" to assert its neurological specificity. While other terms such as Post-Acute Sequelae of SARS-CoV-2 Infection (PASC) remain in use, we argue that PCNS is both clinically and biologically more precise. Our aim in this volume is not only to provide a detailed account of PCNS but to elevate its recognition as a legitimate, measurable, and treatable disorder.

PCNS is best understood not as a single disease but as a syndrome of overlapping mechanisms. These include chronic neuroinflammation, microglial activation, mitochondrial dysfunction, vascular injury, and maladaptive immune responses. The chapters in this book reflect this complexity, with dedicated sections on pathophysiology, biomarkers, cognitive and psychiatric manifestations, autonomic dysfunction, and rehabilitation. Each contributor brings a multidisciplinary perspective, from neurology and epidemiology to rehabilitation sciences and global health.

Importantly, this book is also about people. PCNS has disproportionately affected women, healthcare workers, and individuals in low-resource settings who had limited access to early COVID-19 treatment or vaccination. Health inequity is a recurrent theme. In many low- and middle-income countries (LMICs), the absence of diagnostic infrastructure and specialist care has meant that millions suffer in silence, uncounted and untreated. This is why SDG-3, ensuring healthy lives and promoting well-being for all at all ages, is an ideal framework under which to situate this work.

We are proud to present this volume, and we hope it serves not just as a reference but as a call to action to SDG-3. The scale and diversity of PCNS demand nothing less than global collaboration. Governments, researchers, clinicians, and patient advocacy groups must unite to build surveillance systems, standardize diagnostic tools, fund interdisciplinary trials, and create equitable models of care.

Our journey through this book begins with epidemiological foundations, builds through clinical definitions and mechanistic insights, and culminates in pragmatic solutions for care delivery. Across the volume, we highlight the critical importance of interdisciplinary, culturally informed, and person-centered approaches to PCNS. Whether it is the chapter exploring care delivery and service development or the one focused on patient priorities and narratives, every contribution reminds us that PCNS is not merely a biomedical condition—it is a social, economic, and ethical challenge.

One of the key contributions is the detailed exploration of therapeutic options. The therapeutic chapter offers a comprehensive review of interventions ranging from pharmacological agents like CGRP inhibitors and low-dose naltrexone to neuromodulation and integrative care. It emphasizes the urgent need for multicenter trials and real-world studies that incorporate biomarkers, functional endpoints, and patient-reported outcomes. Importantly, it also advocates for caution—highlighting the risks of therapeutic overreach and unvalidated prescribing patterns seen in many long COVID clinics worldwide.

The chapters on service development and patient needs argue for structured, accessible, and inclusive models of care. They highlight the lived experience of patients and the fragmented nature of current healthcare systems. Their message is clear: without patient-informed care pathways, no amount of research or innovation will translate into real-world impact.

Research needs are addressed head-on, with a call for urgent investment in longitudinal studies, inclusive datasets, and translational partnerships. We must also challenge the research hierarchies that have historically marginalized conditions like PCNS. If we do not address these structural issues, the opportunity to intervene early and meaningfully will be lost.

This book aligns with a broader global movement toward equitable neurological care as articulated in the World Health Organization's Intersectoral Global Action Plan (IGAP) for Epilepsy and Other Neurological Disorders 2022–2031. IGAP represents a milestone in the global neurology landscape. For the first time, a UN health agency has issued a formal action plan calling on Member States to integrate neurological care into universal health coverage and sustainable development policies. PCNS, with its pervasive neurological, cognitive, and psychological impacts, is a quintessential example of a condition that IGAP aims to address—yet it remains missing from many national strategic plans.

WHO's Brain Health Position Paper (2022) further emphasizes the need for life-course, systems-level approaches to brain health. It highlights that neurological disorders are not only the leading cause of disability-adjusted life years (DALYs) globally but also disproportionately affect individuals in low- and middle-income settings. The burden of PCNS adds new urgency to these findings. As millions of people worldwide are now living with persistent post-COVID neurological symptoms, the call for integrated, scalable solutions has never been clearer. By embracing the guiding principles of the brain health framework—access, equity, participation, and accountability—we can begin to move toward more inclusive responses to PCNS.

The IGAP Toolkit, developed by WHO in collaboration with partners including the World Federation of Neurology, offers practical guidance for national and regional implementation of these principles. This book draws inspiration from the toolkit's emphasis on intersectoral collaboration, capacity-building, workforce development, and the inclusion of community and patient voices. PCNS demands precisely this kind of response. The fragmentation of care, the lack of diagnostic clarity, and the marginalization of patient narratives all speak to the need for health systems that are responsive and adaptable. As the IGAP Toolkit suggests, any policy or care model that excludes vulnerable populations or fails to engage primary care will not succeed.

Throughout this volume, readers will find resonances with the five strategic objectives of IGAP:

1. Raise policy priority and strengthen governance
2. Provide effective, timely, and responsive diagnosis, treatment, and care
3. Implement strategies for promotion and prevention
4. Foster research and innovation
5. Strengthen data systems

Each of these pillars is reflected in the structure and intent of this book. Whether through discussions of equitable service delivery, robust surveillance and data needs, or research innovations such as biomarker integration and digital health tools, the goal is the same: to build a foundation for global action against PCNS that is ethically grounded and scientifically robust.

By situating PCNS within the WHO IGAP framework, we amplify its relevance to public health leaders, funders, and global policymakers. We hope this book will serve not just as a clinical and academic resource but as an advocacy tool to secure the recognition and investment that PCNS urgently deserves.

As we conclude this introductory chapter, we reaffirm our commitment to PCNS as a distinct, measurable, and treatable condition. We acknowledge that our knowledge is still evolving, but our intent is clear to build a foundation of scientific integrity, clinical compassion, and global cooperation. We hope this book will inspire researchers, clinicians, and communities to act decisively and inclusively. The work has only just begun.

St. Albans, VIC, Australia Tissa Wijeratne
Seattle, WA, USA Samath Dharmaratne
Nagpur, India Chandrashekar Meshram
St. Albans, VIC, Australia Sheila Crewther

References

1. Davis HE, Assaf GS, McCorkell L, et al. Characterizing Long COVID in an International Cohort: 7 months of symptoms and their impact. EClinicalMedicine 2021;38:101019. https://doi.org/10.1016/j.eclinm.2021.101019.
2. Nalbandian A, Sehgal K, Gupta A, et al. Post-acute COVID-19 syndrome. Nat Med. 2021;27:601–15. https://doi.org/10.1038/s41591-021-01283-z.
3. Oskoui M, Pringsheim T, Billinghurst L, et al. Practice guideline update summary: acute treatment of migraine in children and adolescents: report of the Guideline Development, Dissemination, and Implementation Subcommittee of the American Academy of Neurology and the American Headache Society. Neurology 2019;93(11):487–99. https://doi.org/10.1212/WNL.0000000000008095.
4. Soriano JB, Murthy S, Marshall JC, Relan P, Diaz JV. A clinical case definition of post COVID-19 condition by a Delphi consensus. Lancet Infect Dis. 2022;22(4):e102–7. https://doi.org/10.1016/S1473-3099(21)00703-9.
5. Wijeratne T, Crewther S. Post-COVID-19 Neurological Syndrome (PCNS); A novel syndrome with challenges for the global neurology community. J Neurol Sci. 2020;419:117179. https://doi.org/10.1016/j.jns.2020.117179.
6. World Health Organization. Intersectoral global action plan on epilepsy and other neurological disorders 2022–2031. Geneva: WHO; 2022a. https://www.who.int/publications/i/item/9789240057687.
7. World Health Organization. Position paper: Optimizing brain health across the life course. Geneva: WHO; 2022b. https://www.who.int/publications/i/item/9789240054563.
8. World Health Organization. Toolkit for implementing the intersectoral global action plan on epilepsy and other neurological disorders 2022–2031. Geneva: WHO; 2023. https://www.who.int/publications/i/item/9789240073243.

Contents

1 Global Impact of Post-COVID 19 Neurological Syndrome 1
Chandrashekhar Meshram and Tissa Wijeratne
1.1 Introduction 1
1.2 A Crisis in the Making 1
1.3 The View from the Ground 2
1.4 Why Neurology Must Lead 2
1.5 Aligning with the Sustainable Development Goals 3
1.6 Global Disparities in Brain Health 3
1.7 A Window for Reform 3
1.8 A Call to the Global Neurology Community 4
1.9 What This Chapter Will Explore 4
1.10 Global Impact of Interventions: Vaccination, Education, and Collaboration 4
1.10.1 Vaccination: A Major Public Health Victory 5
1.10.2 Education: Building Awareness and Capacity 5
1.10.3 Collaboration: The Force Multiplier 6
1.11 Real Impact, Real People 6
1.12 The Path Forward 7
1.13 Discussion 7
1.14 Conclusion 9
Further Reading 9

2 Post-COVID-19 Neurological Syndrome: The Epidemiology 11
Reuben Parama Iswara and Tissa Wijeratne
2.1 Introduction 11
2.2 Early Recognition and Historical Perspective 14
2.3 Definition and Characteristics 14
2.4 Mechanisms and Pathophysiology of PCNS 15
2.5 Epidemiology and Prevalence 16
2.5.1 Epidemiology of PCNS in Adults 16
2.5.2 Epidemiology of PCNS in Children and Adolescents 17
2.5.3 Gender Differences in PCNS Prevalence 18
2.5.4 PCNS in Patients with Comorbid Conditions 18

2.5.5 Variability in PCNS Prevalence Due to Study Design and Methodology . . . 18
2.5.6 The Importance of Standardized Definitions and Criteria for PCNS . . . 19
2.5.7 Implications for Public Health and Future Research . . . 19
2.6 Overview of PCNS in Different Populations . . . 20
2.6.1 Demographic and Psychosocial Predictors . . . 20
2.7 Discussion . . . 21
2.8 Conclusion . . . 23
References . . . 23

3 Long-Term Effects of COVID-19 in GBD 2021 . . . 25
Samath Dharmaratne and Tissa Wijeratne
3.1 Introduction . . . 25
3.2 Lived Experiences: Case Snapshots from the Australian Federal Parliament . . . 26
3.2.1 Case 1: Sarah, 38—"I Lost Myself" . . . 26
3.2.2 Case 2: Mark, 45—"It Feels Like My Brain Has Shut Down" . . . 27
3.2.3 Case 3: Priya, 31—"Every Part of My Nervous System is Misfiring" . . . 27
3.2.4 Case 4: Ben, 52—"I'm No Longer the Father I Want to Be" . . . 27
3.2.5 Case 5: Aisha, 29—"I Feel Gaslit by the System" . . . 28
3.2.6 Case 6: Tom, 60—"This Isn't Aging. It's Something Else" . . . 28
3.3 Voices That Demand Recognition . . . 28
3.4 Why Their Stories Matter . . . 28
3.5 Defining PCNS: A Neurological Syndrome . . . 29
3.5.1 Understanding the Full Picture of PCNS Symptoms: What Patients Are Really Living Through . . . 29
3.5.2 Cognitive Impairment and Brain Fog: More Than Just Forgetfulness . . . 30
3.5.3 Memory and Attention Deficits: A Constant Mental Struggle . . . 32
3.5.4 Fatigue . . . 34
3.5.5 Post-COVID Headache: A Key Component of PCNS . . . 36
3.5.6 Sleep and PCNS: A Disrupted Cycle in Neurological Recovery . . . 38
3.5.7 Autonomic Nervous System Dysfunction and PCNS: When the Body's Regulation Breaks Down . . . 40
3.5.8 Understanding the Autonomic Nervous System in PCNS . . . 41
3.6 Postural Orthostatic Tachycardia Syndrome (POTS) . . . 41
3.7 Impact on Daily Life and Function . . . 42

3.8 Diagnostic Challenges and Clinical Misunderstanding 42
3.9 Management Strategies 43
3.10 The Path Forward 43
3.11 Anxiety, Depression, and Emotional Dysregulation: A Secondary Burden, or a Core Symptom? 44
3.11.1 Anxiety: More Than a Reaction 44
3.11.2 Depression and Affective Flattening 45
3.11.3 Emotional Dysregulation: A Neurological Symptom 45
3.11.4 Impact on Identity and Relationships 45
3.11.5 Barriers to Recognition and Care 46
3.11.6 Treatment Considerations 46
3.11.7 Conclusion: Emotion as a Signal, Not a Distraction 46
3.12 Putting It All Together: A Syndrome That Disrupts Identity 47
3.13 Epidemiology and the GBD Framework 47
3.14 Overview of the Global Burden 48
3.15 LMIC-Specific Considerations 48
3.16 Regional Burden and Inequity 49
3.17 Disability and Economic Consequences (Table 3.2) 49
3.18 Why the Name Matters: PCNS Over Long COVID 50
3.19 Recommendations 50
3.20 Conclusion 50
Further Reading 50

4 Post-COVID-19 Neurological Syndrome and the WHO Intersectoral Global Action Plan 53
Reuben Parama Iswara and Tissa Wijeratne
4.1 Policy and Governance Integration: Making PCNS Visible in National Neurological Strategies 55
4.1.1 A Multisystemic Disorder, Requiring Multisectoral Governance 56
4.1.2 Aligning with the Life-Course Approach 56
4.1.3 From National Plans to Funded Action 57
4.1.4 Leveraging Existing Structures and Partnerships 57
4.1.5 Recognizing PCNS in Global Classification Systems 58
4.1.6 Conclusion: Policy Inclusion Is the First Step toward Health Justice 58
4.2 Diagnosis, Treatment, and Care Pathways: From Recognition to Real Response 59
4.2.1 The Care Gap 59
4.2.2 IGAP's Call to Action 60
4.2.3 Diagnostic Challenges and Solutions 60
4.2.4 Treatment and Management Models 61
4.2.5 Scaling the Neurology Workforce 61
4.2.6 A Call for Honesty and Precision 62

4.3 Promotion of Brain Health and Prevention: The Critical Role of Public Awareness and Early Action for PCNS 62
4.3.1 Shifting the Narrative: From "Long COVID" to Brain Health 62
4.3.2 Promoting Brain Health: What We've Already Done 63
4.3.3 Why Prevention Matters for PCNS 64
4.3.4 The Role of Schools, Workplaces, and Primary Care 64
4.3.5 The Role of the Global Burden of Disease (GBD) Study ... 66
4.4 Research: A Neglected Frontier 67
4.4.1 A Health Condition That Strips Away Inclusion 68
4.4.2 The Power of Lived Experience 69
4.4.3 Health Equity and Global Inclusion 70
4.5 Conclusion 72
References 72

5 The Elephant We Refuse to Name: Barriers in PCNS Care 75
Reuben Parama Iswara and Tissa Wijeratne
5.1 Introduction: We Asked. They Answered. But Are We Listening? .. 75
5.2 The Elephant in the Room 76
5.3 A Flood of Fragmented Solutions 76
5.4 What the Scientific Community Is Missing 77
5.5 From Listening to Action 77
5.6 Moving Forward 77
5.7 Understanding the Elephant: Why We Must Do Better Research—With, Not Just on, Patients 78
5.8 A Fractured Landscape 78
5.9 From Participants to Partners 79
5.10 We Need Large, Multidisciplinary Cohorts 79
5.11 Research Must Lead to Change 80
5.12 We Need Urgency and Accountability 80
5.13 Care Fragmentation: Why the Health System Fails to Hold the Whole Patient 81
5.14 Discussion 83
5.15 Conclusion 85
References 85

6 A Call for Services: Building the System PCNS Patients Deserve 87
Shanika Nandasiri and Tissa Wijeratne
6.1 Introduction: We Must Build Together Services, Education, and Research, with Patients at the Center 87
6.2 Services 88
6.3 Education 88
6.4 Research 88
6.5 Walking with Patients and Families 89
6.6 The Time Is Now 89

6.7 Building the First Pillar: Services that Truly Support People with PCNS 90
6.8 What Does a PCNS Service Look Like 90
6.9 Key Features of Effective PCNS Services 90
6.10 Learning from Other Conditions 91
6.11 Why It Matters 91
6.12 What Patients Are Telling Us 91
6.13 Moving Forward 92
6.14 Training Clinicians at Every Level 92
6.15 Medical and Allied Health Curricula 93
6.16 Educating the Public 93
6.17 Supporting Families and Carers 94
6.18 Learning from the Patients Themselves 94
6.19 From Knowledge to Action 95
6.20 Building the Third Pillar: Research that Leads to Real Solutions . . . 95
6.21 The Case for Research Urgency 95
6.22 What Kind of Research Do We Need 96
6.23 Research Must Be Patient-Led 96
6.24 Funding and Coordination 97
6.25 Moving from Discovery to Impact 97
6.26 The Role of the IGAP Framework 97
6.27 Discussion 98
6.28 Conclusion 99
References 99

7 Education in Post-COVID Neurological Syndrome (PCNS) 101
Vimukthi Pathiraja, Tissa Wijeratne, and Reuben Parama Iswara
7.1 Introduction: Why Education Is Central to the Future of PCNS Care 101
7.2 Understanding the Educational Imperative for PCNS 103
7.3 Early Detection and Diagnosis 105
7.4 Recognizing Early Symptoms 105
7.5 Diagnostic Tools and Clinical Evaluation 106
7.6 Bringing Early Detection into the Real World 107
7.7 Involving Patients in Diagnostic Education 107
7.8 Comprehensive Patient Management 107
7.9 Educational Needs for Healthcare Professionals 108
7.10 Educational Requirements in Low-Income Settings 109
7.11 Utilizing Community Health Workers 110
7.12 Distance Learning and Technology-Based Solutions 111
7.13 Educational Requirements in High-Income Settings 111
7.14 Advanced Training Programs 111
7.15 Research and Evidence-Based Practice 112
7.16 Interdisciplinary Collaboration in PCNS Education 113
7.17 Communication Skills Development in PCNS Education 114

7.18 Challenges in Implementing PCNS Education . . . 116
7.19 Language and Cultural Barriers . . . 117
7.20 Need for Political and Institutional Support . . . 117
7.21 Future Directions: Building Stronger PCNS Education . . . 117
7.22 Future Directions and Conclusion . . . 118
7.22.1 Expanding Digital Learning Platforms . . . 118
7.22.2 Building Collaborative Networks . . . 118
7.22.3 Continuous Evaluation and Improvement . . . 119
7.23 Final Thoughts . . . 119
Further Reading . . . 120

8 Research Needs in Post-COVID Neurological Syndrome . . . 123
Tissa Wijeratne and Sheila Crewther
8.1 Introduction—Rethinking Research for Post-COVID Neurological Syndrome . . . 123
8.2 Recognizing the Urgency: A Systems Level Call to Action for Post-COVID Neurological Syndrome . . . 125
8.3 Discussion . . . 129
References . . . 132

9 Therapeutic Options for Post-COVID 19 Neurological Syndrome . . . 133
Reuben Parama Iswara and Tissa Wijeratne
9.1 Introduction . . . 133
9.2 Discussion: The Path Forward for Therapeutic Research in Post-COVID-19 Neurological Syndrome (PCNS) . . . 142
References . . . 145

10 Patient Needs in PCNS Care . . . 147
Reuben Parama Iswara and Tissa Wijeratne
10.1 Introduction . . . 147
10.2 Recognition and Diagnostic Legitimacy . . . 149
10.3 Accessible and Coordinated Care Pathways . . . 150
10.4 Psychological and Emotional Support . . . 152
10.5 Socioeconomic Protection and Workplace Accommodations . . . 154
10.6 Inclusion of Lived Experience in Policy and Research Design . . . 157
10.7 Discussion and Conclusion . . . 159
References . . . 161

11 Brain Fog in the Young Insights from a Meta-analytic Review of Cognitive Impairment in Pediatric PCNS . . . 163
Melanie J. Murphy, Lauren Falcone, and Nina Riddell
11.1 Introduction . . . 163
11.2 Methods . . . 164
11.3 Findings and Interpretation . . . 165
11.3.1 Prevalence of Cognitive Impairments in Pediatric PASC . . 165

11.4 Theoretical and Clinical Implications 166
11.4.1 Complex Attention as a Core Deficit 166
11.4.2 The Role of Memory and Executive Function 167
11.4.3 Dose-Response and Risk Stratification 167
11.4.4 Parallels with CFS/ME and a Systems-Based View 167
11.4.5 Limitations and Gaps in the Literature 168
11.4.6 Educational and Clinical Implications 168
11.4.7 Standardizing Post-COVID Cognitive Screening 169
11.4.8 Understanding the Whole Child 169
11.5 Conclusion 169
References 170

12 Long Covid or Post-Covid -19 Neurological Syndrome? 175
Tissa Wijeratne and Sheila Crewther
12.1 Introduction 175
12.2 Framing the Clinical Case for PCNS 177
12.3 Data Driven Arguments and Emerging Biological Evidence 178
12.4 Implications for Care, Research, and Health Policy 183
References 185

13 Post-COVID Neurological Syndrome: A Turning Point for Brain Health and Sustainable Development 187
Tissa Wijeratne and Sheila Crewther
13.1 Introduction 187
13.2 What We Tried to Say in This Book 189
13.3 What Did We Cover? 190
13.4 PCNS, Brain Health, and SDG 3: A Shared Crisis, a Shared Opportunity 191
13.5 What Does PCNS Share with Headache Disorders? 192
13.6 Where Does SDG 3 Come In? 192
13.7 The Power of Framing PCNS as a Development Issue 193
13.8 What Would Success Look Like? 193
13.9 We Know What to Do 194
13.10 A Shared Message Across All Chapters 194
13.11 Conclusion 195
13.12 What Do We Hope to Achieve? 195
13.13 In Closing 196
Further Reading 196

Global Impact of Post-COVID 19 Neurological Syndrome

1

Chandrashekhar Meshram and Tissa Wijeratne

1.1 Introduction

The world is living through the largest neurological crisis of the twenty first century.

Post-COVID 19 neurological syndrome, or PCNS, is real. It is disabling, and it is affecting millions of people around the globe. It has emerged as one of the most significant long-term consequences of the COVID 19 pandemic. PCNS is not just a lingering viral effect. It is a complex, multisystem neurological condition that disrupts memory, attention, mood, sleep, movement, and autonomic function. It does not follow borders. It does not respect income levels, and yet, it remains dangerously under recognized.

We are now more than 4 years into the pandemic. Despite the shift in public focus, the long shadow of SARS CoV 2 continues, and in that shadow are millions of people who are struggling. They are not recovering. They are not being heard. This chapter sets the stage for why that matters—not just to neurology, but to global health, economic recovery, and the future of inclusive development.

1.2 A Crisis in the Making

PCNS affects up to 30%–40% of individuals who recover from COVID 19. That is hundreds of millions of people worldwide. The symptoms vary but are often invisible to standard tests. Brain fog. Headache. Fatigue. Numbness. Mood changes.

C. Meshram (✉)
Brain and Mind Institute, Nagpur, India

AIIMS, Bibinagar, Hyderabad, India

T. Wijeratne
Department of Neurology and Stroke, La Trobe University, St. Albans, VIC, Australia
e-mail: tissa.wijeratne@wh.org.au

T. Wijeratne, S. Crewther (eds.), *Post Covid-19 Neurological Syndrome*,
https://doi.org/10.1007/978-3-032-14995-4_1

Sleep disturbance. Difficulty returning to work or school. These symptoms affect function, quality of life, and long term health outcomes.

The burden is disproportionately high in low- and middle-income countries. These are the places where testing is limited, follow up care is rare, and neurological expertise is scarce. PCNS adds pressure to already stretched health systems. It worsens existing inequities, and it risks creating a second pandemic of brain-based disability.

1.3 The View from the Ground

In high income countries, patients with PCNS may be referred to long COVID clinics or specialist teams. In contrast, in many lower income settings, there are no such options. People are told they are anxious. They are ignored, or worse, they are blamed. As clinicians working in these settings, we have seen the cost: Mothers who cannot care for their children, health workers who cannot return to their jobs, students who cannot finish their studies, farmers and laborers who cannot manage their daily activities.

PCNS does not just affect the brain. It affects families, communities, and economies.

1.4 Why Neurology Must Lead

This is a neurological emergency. The brain is the organ most commonly affected in the post-COVID phase. We must stop treating this as a vague post-viral illness. The evidence is now overwhelming. PCNS is a brain condition driven by chronic low grade inflammation, neuroimmune activation, and disrupted brain networks. It is time for the global neurology community to lead.

The World Federation of Neurology (WFN) has long been a voice for brain health. Since 2014, WFN has led the World Brain Day campaign to bring attention to the most urgent issues in neurological care. Each year, the campaign reaches over 1 billion people. The 2025 theme—*Brain Health for All Ages*—could not be more timely. PCNS affects children, adults, and older people. It is the clearest example of why lifelong brain health must be a global goal.

WFN's vision aligns closely with the World Health Organization's Intersectoral Global Action Plan (IGAP) on Epilepsy and Other Neurological Disorders. IGAP is a bold strategy that calls for neurological conditions to be integrated into national health plans, with attention to equity, access, and capacity building. PCNS fits every part of that plan.

1.5 Aligning with the Sustainable Development Goals

PCNS is not just a health issue. It is a development issue. It strikes hardest at those already vulnerable: Women, people with disabilities, the unemployed, migrant workers, children in poor schools, people in rural areas. It is a challenge that sits at the intersection of many of the United Nations Sustainable Development Goals (SDGs).

- *SDG 3* calls for good health and wellbeing at all ages. PCNS directly threatens that goal.
- *SDG 5* calls for gender equality. Women are disproportionately affected by PCNS, yet often dismissed.
- *SDG 8* calls for decent work and economic growth. PCNS impairs employment and productivity.
- *SDG 10* demands reduced inequalities, but PCNS deepens them. Especially in places with no access to neurology care.

If we do not act on PCNS, we will not meet our global development goals. The damage will not be seen only in hospital records. It will be seen in classrooms, workplaces, and homes.

1.6 Global Disparities in Brain Health

The world already faces major disparities in neurological care. According to WHO, more than 40% of countries have fewer than one neurologist per 100,000 people. In many African and South Asian nations, that number is closer to one per million. Most people with epilepsy, stroke, or dementia in these settings receive no specialist care. PCNS adds to this burden. Without action, it will overwhelm already fragile systems.

It is essential that PCNS be included in global brain health strategies. We cannot wait years for consensus definitions and randomized trials before we act. The science is evolving, but the suffering is already here.

1.7 A Window for Reform

COVID 19 has exposed the weaknesses of our health systems, but it has also opened a window for reform. Governments are paying attention. People understand more about immunity, inflammation, and recovery than ever before. We must seize this moment.

PCNS gives us a chance to build something better: A new model of care that is brain focused, community based, and person centered; A new research agenda that includes low resource settings from the start; A new approach to education that empowers primary care and community health workers; A new public conversation about brain health and recovery.

1.8 A Call to the Global Neurology Community

We cannot address PCNS in isolation, but we also cannot ignore it. The global neurology community must take leadership now. That means:

- Advocating for the inclusion of PCNS in national neurology and rehabilitation strategies
- Partnering with ministries of health to build care models that include PCNS
- Training the next generation of clinicians in post-viral brain syndromes
- Collaborating across borders to build registries, share data, and learn together
- Engaging patients and caregivers as partners in research and service design

The WFN, WHO, and other global partners have laid the groundwork. IGAP gives us the roadmap. The SDGs give us the motivation. World Brain Day gives us the platform. Now we must deliver the solutions.

1.9 What This Chapter Will Explore

In the sections that follow, we will examine the global data on PCNS. We will describe how it presents across different regions. We will explore its social and economic costs. We will focus especially on low and middle income countries where resources are limited, but the burden is rising fast.

We will argue that PCNS is a defining issue for modern neurology, and we will show that by recognizing and responding to it, we can transform not only patient lives, but the way we understand and support brain health across the globe.

This is the moment to act. The science is strong. The voices are loud. The need is clear. PCNS is a global issue. Neurology must meet it with a global response.

1.10 Global Impact of Interventions: Vaccination, Education, and Collaboration

While the burden of Post-COVID 19 Neurological Syndrome (PCNS) continues to grow, we are not without tools to fight back. The global response to COVID 19 has already demonstrated the incredible power of science, public health infrastructure, education, and international collaboration. Now, we must extend those lessons to PCNS.

1.10.1 Vaccination: A Major Public Health Victory

One of the most powerful weapons in our arsenal has been vaccination. COVID 19 vaccines have saved millions of lives, but their value extends beyond acute infection. Emerging evidence suggests that vaccination also reduces the risk and severity of PCNS.

People who are vaccinated before infection are less likely to develop long-term neurological symptoms. Even those vaccinated after recovery may see improvements in fatigue and brain fog. This is not only a clinical gain—it is a global economic and social advantage.

However, in many low and middle income countries, vaccination coverage remains uneven. Logistics, misinformation, and supply chain barriers persist. Increasing vaccine access, especially in rural and marginalized communities, is critical—not just to prevent acute COVID 19 but to mitigate long term brain health impacts.

We must frame vaccine equity as brain health equity. International donors, governments, and advocacy groups need to include PCNS outcomes in their vaccine campaigns. It is not only about saving lives. It is also about saving minds, livelihoods, and futures.

1.10.2 Education: Building Awareness and Capacity

Education is a second pillar of our global response. COVID 19 has transformed public understanding of science, immunity, and health risks, but when it comes to PCNS, misinformation and confusion remain widespread.

Patients are often misdiagnosed or dismissed. Clinicians are unsure how to assess or manage symptoms. Policymakers do not recognize the scale of the problem. We must fix this.

Medical curricula must be updated. PCNS should be part of neurology, internal medicine, rehabilitation, and primary care training. Nurses, physiotherapists, occupational therapists, and mental health workers all need knowledge of PCNS. In low and middle income countries, where specialists are few, this is especially important.

Community education is also essential. Patients need access to plain-language information. Schools and workplaces need policies to accommodate people with cognitive and physical fatigue. Mass media campaigns can play a role. Social media, if used responsibly, can amplify the voices of patients and support networks.

Education empowers patients to advocate for themselves. It equips providers to care more effectively. It helps families and caregivers understand what is happening. It shifts blame away from the individual and toward a shared responsibility for care and recovery.

1.10.3 Collaboration: The Force Multiplier

Global collaboration has always been the backbone of effective health responses. During COVID 19, we saw unprecedented levels of knowledge sharing. Researchers published data in real time. Countries shared protocols and strategies. Organizations coordinated vaccine rollouts. This same model must now be applied to PCNS.

We need multinational studies, shared registries, unified definitions, collaborative trials, open access to data, and global funding pools. No one country or institution can do this alone.

The World Health Organization's Intersectoral Global Action Plan on Neurological Disorders provides a perfect platform. It calls for integrated care, workforce development, better surveillance, and stronger partnerships. PCNS belongs at the heart of this plan.

The World Federation of Neurology has already led the way through the World Brain Day campaign. The 2025 theme, "Brain Health for All Ages," offers a unique opportunity to highlight PCNS in a global context. National neurological societies, patient advocacy groups, and civil society organizations should join forces to use this platform to push for change.

South South collaborations should be expanded. Knowledge must flow not just from high income to low income countries, but in both directions. Community based solutions developed in Africa, South Asia, or Latin America may hold keys to effective, scalable PCNS care.

Cross discipline collaboration is also key. Neurologists must work with immunologists, rehabilitation experts, psychologists, public health professionals, and patients. PCNS is not a single system disease. It is a complex, dynamic, evolving condition that demands holistic thinking.

1.11 Real Impact, Real People

The benefits of these interventions are not theoretical. They change lives. A vaccinated teacher who avoids brain fog can keep her job. A trained primary care nurse in a remote clinic can recognize PCNS early and prevent disability. A collaborative research study can discover a new therapy that brings relief to millions.

In Sri Lanka, an education campaign led to early referrals and better outcomes. In Uganda, mobile clinics supported by WHO reached thousands of people with suspected PCNS. In Brazil, online rehabilitation groups helped patients manage fatigue and anxiety. In Australia, patient led advocacy groups are shaping care pathways and funding priorities.

Each of these examples shows that with the right tools and partnerships, change is possible. Even in the most resource constrained settings, impact can be achieved.

1.12 The Path Forward

Vaccination, education, and collaboration are not luxury strategies. They are essential, and they are feasible, even in low income contexts, but they require political will, community trust, and long term vision.

We must move from short term emergency responses to sustainable, system wide planning. PCNS is not going away, but with the right approach, we can reduce its burden, improve recovery, and protect brain health globally.

It is time to think bigger. To act bolder, and to work together, across borders, across disciplines, and across generations.

If we do, we will not only meet the challenge of PCNS. We will build a stronger, fairer, more resilient future for brain health worldwide.

1.13 Discussion

The emergence of Post-COVID 19 Neurological Syndrome (PCNS) has shifted the landscape of global neurology. What began as scattered clinical observations has now solidified into a large-scale neurological challenge affecting millions across all regions of the world. The symptoms of PCNS are now well-documented—fatigue, cognitive decline, autonomic dysfunction, mood disturbance, and sensory changes, but despite the growing scientific understanding, the global response remains fragmented. This discussion highlights the key challenges and opportunities in addressing PCNS through the lens of equity, systems thinking, and global health.

One of the most striking aspects of PCNS is its wide reach. It affects people of all ages and backgrounds, yet the degree of suffering is not equally shared. People living in low and middle income countries bear the highest burden. This is not due to a biological difference. It is due to disparities in access, education, and care. In many settings, even recognizing PCNS is a challenge. Diagnostic tools are unavailable. Specialists are scarce. Rehabilitation services are underfunded, and the stigma around invisible symptoms leads to widespread dismissal of patient complaints.

Moreover, PCNS exposes a critical weakness in global health systems. Neurology has long been underfunded and underprioritized. According to the World Health Organization, most countries still do not have a dedicated national strategy for neurological disorders. This is despite the fact that neurological conditions are the second leading cause of death and the leading cause of disability worldwide. PCNS must now act as a wake-up call for health systems to invest in brain health infrastructure from data collection to service delivery and workforce training.

The World Federation of Neurology (WFN) has played a leading role in raising global awareness. Since 2014, the World Brain Day campaign has reached over a billion people with messages of brain health advocacy and inclusion. The 2025 theme, *Brain Health for All Ages*, is especially relevant to PCNS. It reminds us that neurological care should not be limited to older adults or stroke survivors. It must include children with learning delays, working adults with brain fog, and elderly people struggling with post-viral fatigue.

Global collaboration will be essential. No single country or organization can solve PCNS alone. We must build global registries, harmonize diagnostic criteria, share data, and learn from diverse models of care. This includes lessons from previous neuroinfections such as Japanese encephalitis, Zika, or HIV-associated cognitive disorders. Low resource settings have rich experience in community-based neurology, mobile care, and task-shifting strategies. These approaches must now be adapted to PCNS.

Vaccination remains one of the most effective interventions. Studies consistently show that people vaccinated before infection have lower rates of PCNS. This highlights an important policy link—improving vaccine access is not only about reducing hospitalizations or death. It is about protecting long-term brain function. However, vaccination alone is not enough. Patients who develop PCNS still need comprehensive, multidisciplinary support.

Digital health tools present a promising opportunity. Smartphone-based cognitive tests, tele-rehabilitation, and AI-supported symptom tracking can help scale access to care, particularly in rural or underserved communities, but digital solutions must be accompanied by efforts to ensure digital literacy, privacy, and cultural relevance. Technology cannot replace the human need for empathy, time, and continuity of care.

Another key issue is research. PCNS remains under-researched relative to its global burden. Most studies come from high-income countries and focus on adult populations. We need more inclusive research that spans age groups, languages, and cultures. We also need better biological markers to diagnose PCNS objectively and track recovery. Funding agencies must prioritize PCNS as a critical area for investment, and journals must provide platforms for diverse voices and perspectives.

Mental health integration is vital. PCNS often overlaps with depression, anxiety, trauma, and grief. These are not separate conditions but part of the same post-viral syndrome affecting brain circuits. Integrated mental health and neurological care can reduce fragmentation and stigma. Community-based counselling, peer support, and culturally sensitive psychological care can play a crucial role in recovery.

Workplace policies must also adapt. Many people with PCNS are unable to return to full-time work or require flexible schedules. Employers and governments must collaborate to develop guidelines for return-to-work planning, disability support, and workplace accommodations. Without these supports, PCNS becomes a pathway to poverty, unemployment, and social exclusion.

Importantly, the voice of the patient must guide all these efforts. Lived experience is not an optional add-on. It is central to building trust, designing relevant services, and measuring meaningful outcomes. Patient-led organizations have already shown how powerful storytelling, advocacy, and co-design can be. These efforts must be recognized, supported, and institutionalized.

In summary, the global impact of PCNS is far-reaching, but not unmanageable. It will require us to reimagine how we think about brain health moving from episodic care to lifelong support, from high-tech to high-touch, and from exclusion to inclusion. The tools exist. The knowledge is growing. What is needed now is political will, coordinated action, and a shared global vision.

1.14 Conclusion

Post-COVID 19 Neurological Syndrome is a global challenge that demands a global response. It is a condition that has brought new urgency to the field of neurology. Millions of people across the world are living with the daily consequences of PCNS—memory problems, fatigue, pain, disorientation, and loss of identity. These symptoms are not invisible to those who live with them. They are deeply felt, deeply disruptive, and often life-altering.

This chapter has highlighted the scale and complexity of the problem. PCNS is not only a health issue. It is a development issue. It touches on education, employment, mental health, and social justice. It disproportionately affects women, front-line workers, migrants, and people in low-resource settings. These are the same populations that are often left behind in healthcare systems that were never built for chronic, complex, and poorly understood conditions.

We have also highlighted solutions. Vaccination, education, digital tools, workforce training, mental health integration, and community-based care models are all feasible. They are already making a difference in parts of the world. What is missing is scale, investment, and political commitment. PCNS needs to be named, funded, and prioritized in global and national health strategies. It must be included in the WHO's IGAP implementation plans and directly linked to achieving SDG 3 and related development goals.

Above all, we must remember that behind the numbers are people. People who were healthy before the pandemic. People who want to work, to learn, to connect, and to thrive. People who deserve care, recognition, and hope.

This is not the end of the pandemic story. It is the beginning of a new chapter in global brain health. Let us make it one defined not by neglect, but by action. Not by silence, but by solidarity.

Let this be the decade we changed what it means to recover.

Further Reading

Wijeratne T, Crewther S. Post-COVID 19 neurological syndrome (PCNS); a novel syndrome with challenges for the global neurology community. J Neurol Sci. 2020;419:117179. https://doi.org/10.1016/j.jns.2020.117179.

Davis HE, Assaf GS, McCorkell L, et al. Characterizing long COVID in an international cohort: 7 months of symptoms and their impact. EClinicalMedicine. 2021;38:101019. https://doi.org/10.1016/j.eclinm.2021.101019.

Taquet M, Geddes JR, Husain M, et al. 6-month neurological and psychiatric outcomes in 236,379 survivors of COVID-19. Lancet Psychiatry. 2021;8(5):416–27. https://doi.org/10.1016/S2215-0366(21)00084-5.

United Nations. Transforming our world: the 2030 agenda for sustainable development. 2015. Available at: https://sdgs.un.org/goals/goal3. Accessed 18 May 2025.

World Federation of Neurology. World brain day 2025: brain health for all ages. 2024. Available at: https://wfneurology.org/world-brain-day. Accessed 18 May 2025.

World Health Organization. Intersectoral global action plan on epilepsy and other neurological disorders 2022–2031. Geneva: WHO; 2022.

World Health Organization. Brain health: optimizing brain health across the life course. Geneva: WHO; 2023.

Graham EL, et al. Persistent neurologic symptoms and cognitive dysfunction in non-hospitalized COVID-19 long haulers. Ann Clin Transl Neurol. 2021;8(5):1073–85.

Rajan S, et al. Policy brief: long COVID—preparing for the long haul. WHO Europe; 2021.

Nasserie T, Hittle M, Goodman SN. Assessment of persistent symptoms among patients with COVID-19: a systematic review. JAMA Netw Open. 2021;4(5):e2111417.

GBD 2019 Diseases and Injuries Collaborators. Global burden of 369 diseases and injuries in 204 countries and territories. Lancet. 2020;396(10258):1204–22.

Sudre CH, et al. Attributes and predictors of long COVID. Nat Med. 2021;27(4):626–31.

Carfi A, Bernabei R, Landi F. Persistent symptoms in patients after acute COVID-19. JAMA. 2020;324(6):603–5.

Nalbandian A, et al. Post-acute COVID-19 syndrome. Nat Med. 2021;27:601–15.

Ceban F, et al. Fatigue and cognitive impairment in post COVID-19 syndrome. Brain Behav Immun Health. 2022;19:100461.

Lopez-Leon S, et al. More than 50 long-term effects of COVID-19. Sci Rep. 2021;11:16144.

Aamodt AH, et al. Comorbidity of headache and psychiatric disorders. J Headache Pain. 2006;7(4):210–9.

Zubair AS, et al. Neuropathogenesis and neurologic manifestations of COVID-19. JAMA Neurol. 2020;77(8):1018–27.

World Health Organization. Headache disorders and public health: education and management implications. Geneva: WHO; 2016.

Institute for Health Metrics and Evaluation (IHME). Global burden of disease study 2021 (GBD 2021). Seattle: IHME; 2022.

Post-COVID-19 Neurological Syndrome: The Epidemiology

2

Reuben Parama Iswara and Tissa Wijeratne

2.1 Introduction

The global spread of COVID-19 has brought about an unprecedented public health crisis, impacting virtually every country and altering the lives of millions. Since its emergence in late 2019, the SARS-CoV-2 virus, which causes COVID-19, has been primarily characterized by its respiratory and systemic effects. The rapid spread, high transmissibility, and severity of COVID-19 have placed a significant strain on healthcare systems, leading to an intense focus on managing the acute symptoms of the virus. These symptoms predominantly include fever, cough, difficulty breathing, and, in severe cases, respiratory failure, pneumonia, and multi-organ dysfunction. However, as the pandemic continues, it has become clear that the impact of COVID-19 extends far beyond the acute phase of infection. Many COVID-19 survivors experience prolonged and, in some cases, debilitating symptoms that persist long after recovery. Among these long-term effects, a growing body of evidence points to significant neurological and cognitive sequelae collectively known as Post-COVID Neurological Syndrome (PCNS).

Post-COVID Neurological Syndrome (PCNS) encompasses a wide array of neurological symptoms that persist or emerge after the initial infection has subsided. This syndrome represents a complex and often disabling condition that affects the nervous system, manifesting as cognitive impairment, sensory disturbances, autonomic dysfunction, persistent fatigue, and mood changes. For many individuals, PCNS severely affects quality of life, limiting their ability to work, socialize, and

R. Parama Iswara (✉)
Department of Neurology, Western Health, Melbourne, VIC, Australia
e-mail: Reuben.ParamaIswara@wh.org.au

T. Wijeratne
Department of Neurology and Stroke, La Trobe University, St. Albans, VIC, Australia
e-mail: tissa.wijeratne@wh.org.au

T. Wijeratne, S. Crewther (eds.), *Post Covid-19 Neurological Syndrome*,
https://doi.org/10.1007/978-3-032-14995-4_2

engage in normal daily activities. PCNS affects not only those who experienced severe COVID-19, requiring hospitalization or intensive care, but also individuals who had mild or even asymptomatic cases. This widespread occurrence across diverse populations suggests that PCNS is not solely a consequence of severe respiratory illness but may be directly related to the virus's impact on the nervous system.

While the phenomenon of long-term symptoms following viral infections is not new—historically, conditions like chronic fatigue syndrome and post-viral encephalitis have been associated with viral infections—COVID-19's sheer global reach has rendered PCNS a distinct public health challenge. The wide-ranging nature of PCNS symptoms has drawn attention to the syndrome as a unique entity with broad implications for both individual patients and healthcare systems. This complexity arises not only from the diversity of symptoms but also from the overlapping mechanisms involved, including neuroinflammation, immune dysregulation, mitochondrial dysfunction, and possible vascular and microvascular damage.

The emergence of PCNS represents a significant shift in how long-term sequelae of COVID-19 are understood and managed. The medical community is familiar with post-viral syndromes, yet the scope and impact of PCNS are unprecedented due to the COVID-19 pandemic's scale and the large number of individuals affected. Researchers, clinicians, and policymakers now face the formidable challenge of understanding, diagnosing, and managing a syndrome that is both heterogeneous and evolving. Unlike many post-viral syndromes, PCNS appears to involve multiple systems within the body, affecting the central and peripheral nervous systems, cardiovascular system, and immune system. Symptoms are diverse, ranging from cognitive dysfunction and "brain fog" to neuropathic pain, loss of smell, gastrointestinal symptoms, and autonomic instability. The multitude of symptoms poses a diagnostic challenge, as they can vary in severity, appear in isolation or clusters, and overlap with other medical and psychiatric conditions.

Understanding PCNS also involves addressing significant knowledge gaps in its epidemiology and pathophysiology. Early studies suggest that up to 50% of COVID-19 survivors may experience at least one neurological or cognitive symptom related to PCNS. These estimates, however, are challenging to standardize due to varying definitions of PCNS, differences in study design, and diverse patient populations. Furthermore, the prevalence and severity of symptoms appear to vary widely depending on factors such as age, gender, pre-existing health conditions, and the severity of the initial infection. Younger, previously healthy individuals have reported disabling PCNS symptoms, highlighting that even those with mild COVID-19 cases are at risk. This unpredictability complicates efforts to identify high-risk individuals and underscores the need for systematic research to establish consistent diagnostic criteria, risk factors, and prognostic indicators for PCNS.

The long-term nature of PCNS and its widespread occurrence among COVID-19 survivors place additional demands on healthcare systems already stretched by the pandemic. The ongoing need for follow-up care, neurological assessments, cognitive rehabilitation, and mental health support has highlighted substantial gaps in healthcare infrastructure. For healthcare systems that were initially focused on managing acute COVID-19 cases, the shift toward addressing chronic conditions such as PCNS requires significant adaptation. Neurology and mental health services, in particular, face increasing demands, as PCNS patients often require comprehensive, multidisciplinary care. The economic impact of PCNS is also substantial, as prolonged symptoms can result in lost productivity, increased healthcare costs, and, for some individuals, long-term disability.

One of the core challenges of PCNS lies in its diagnostic complexity. The syndrome lacks a universally accepted definition and standardized diagnostic criteria, leading to variability in diagnosis and management. Symptoms such as memory impairment, difficulty concentrating, and persistent fatigue are often subtle and may be overlooked or misattributed to psychological distress, burnout, or other unrelated conditions. For example, "brain fog," a commonly reported symptom of PCNS, is characterized by a subjective sense of mental cloudiness, slower thinking, and difficulty with memory and focus. These cognitive complaints can be debilitating yet are challenging to quantify using traditional neurocognitive testing. Similarly, autonomic symptoms, such as heart palpitations, orthostatic intolerance, and blood pressure fluctuations, may not be immediately linked to COVID-19, especially in patients with mild initial infections. The lack of specific biomarkers or diagnostic tests for PCNS further complicates identification, leading to potential delays in treatment and management.

The pathophysiology of PCNS is an area of active research, with multiple theories being explored to explain the diverse neurological manifestations observed in COVID-19 survivors. One prominent hypothesis is that neuroinflammation plays a central role, with SARS-CoV-2 triggering an immune response that affects the brain and nervous system. The "cytokine storm" associated with severe COVID-19 cases is thought to increase blood-brain barrier permeability, allowing inflammatory cytokines and immune cells to infiltrate the brain. This inflammatory response can activate microglial cells, leading to neural damage and potential long-term cognitive and psychological effects. Another theory focuses on mitochondrial dysfunction, as SARS-CoV-2 has been shown to disrupt mitochondrial function, potentially leading to energy deficits in neurons and muscle cells. This disruption could account for the profound fatigue and cognitive symptoms reported in PCNS patients.

Another emerging area of research involves autonomic and microvascular dysfunction, as SARS-CoV-2 appears to damage the endothelium of blood vessels, leading to impaired blood flow in the brain and other organs. This microvascular damage could contribute to symptoms such as orthostatic intolerance, dizziness, and sensory disturbances seen in PCNS. Understanding these pathophysiological mechanisms is essential for developing targeted therapeutic interventions that address the root causes of PCNS rather than merely alleviating symptoms. However, much remains to be learned, and ongoing research is critical to establish effective treatment protocols.

The widespread prevalence and impact of PCNS underscore the urgent need for healthcare adaptation and policy action. Addressing PCNS effectively requires a coordinated, multidisciplinary approach that encompasses medical, neurological, psychological, and rehabilitative care. Primary care providers, neurologists, psychiatrists, and rehabilitation specialists all play critical roles in managing PCNS, necessitating increased training and resources to recognize and treat this condition effectively. Public health initiatives are also essential to increase awareness of PCNS, reduce stigma, and encourage COVID-19 survivors to seek care for persistent symptoms. Policy measures, such as funding for research, the establishment of specialized PCNS clinics, and support for long-term disability, are vital to supporting affected individuals and reducing the syndrome's economic impact.

In summary, Post-COVID Neurological Syndrome represents a profound shift in the understanding of COVID-19's long-term effects. The syndrome poses complex challenges to the medical and scientific communities, given its heterogeneous symptoms, unclear diagnostic criteria, and evolving pathophysiology. The impact of PCNS is significant not only for individual patients but also for healthcare systems and society at large. Addressing PCNS requires a comprehensive approach that includes epidemiological research, healthcare adaptation, therapeutic development, and policy support. As the global health community grapples with the pandemic's ongoing legacy, prioritizing research and resources for PCNS is essential to improve quality of life for millions of COVID-19 survivors and to develop a robust response to this emerging public health crisis.

2.2 Early Recognition and Historical Perspective

In the early months of the COVID-19 pandemic, clinicians worldwide began to report neurological symptoms in patients who had otherwise recovered from the acute phase of infection [1]. Initial cases predominantly involved patients who had been hospitalized or required intensive care, but soon, neurological complaints were also observed in those who experienced mild or asymptomatic infections. These symptoms, which ranged from cognitive deficits and memory issues to fatigue and headaches, persisted well beyond the resolution of respiratory and systemic symptoms, indicating a possible long-term impact of SARS-CoV-2 on the nervous system.

The concept of post-viral syndromes is not entirely new. Historical examples, such as chronic fatigue syndrome following Epstein-Barr virus infection and neurological complications after influenza, laid the foundation for understanding how viral infections can lead to persistent neurological sequelae. However, the scale and diversity of symptoms associated with PCNS are unparalleled, driven by the global reach and high transmissibility of SARS-CoV-2. The persistence of these symptoms, coupled with the sheer number of individuals affected by COVID-19, has transformed PCNS into a major public health concern, underscoring the need for a coordinated response to address its unique challenges.

2.3 Definition and Characteristics

PCNS refers to a collection of symptoms that persist beyond the acute phase of COVID-19 and affect the central and peripheral nervous systems. These symptoms vary widely, but commonly reported manifestations include cognitive impairment, often termed "brain fog," sensory changes such as loss of smell (anosmia) or altered taste (dysgeusia), autonomic instability, chronic fatigue, mood disturbances, and neuropathic pain. PCNS can develop irrespective of the initial infection severity, impacting individuals who experienced mild, moderate, or severe COVID-19, as well as those with asymptomatic infections.

The diverse presentation of PCNS symptoms has complicated efforts to establish consistent diagnostic criteria. Researchers are working to categorize PCNS subtypes based on symptomatology, duration, and underlying pathophysiological mechanisms. Current definitions of PCNS are broad and encompass a range of post-COVID conditions, including Long COVID and Post-Acute COVID Syndrome (PACS). As scientific understanding of PCNS grows, it is increasingly recognized that the syndrome may share mechanistic features with other post-infectious and chronic inflammatory conditions, suggesting potential avenues for treatment and intervention.

2.4 Mechanisms and Pathophysiology of PCNS

Neuroinflammation is thought to be a primary driver of PCNS symptoms. During acute COVID-19, the body mounts a strong immune response to the SARS-CoV-2 virus, leading to the release of inflammatory markers such as cytokines (e.g., IL-6, IL-1β, TNF-α). This cytokine response can be extreme, particularly in severe cases, culminating in a "cytokine storm." The blood-brain barrier, normally a robust shield for the CNS, can become compromised by inflammatory mediators, allowing cytokines and immune cells to infiltrate the brain.

Microglial cells, the brain's resident immune cells, may become activated by this immune response, leading to sustained neuroinflammation. While acute activation of microglia is a natural immune response, chronic activation can damage neural cells and disrupt neural circuits, contributing to cognitive deficits and mood disturbances commonly observed in PCNS. Understanding the pathways of neuroinflammation and finding ways to modulate microglial activity are active areas of research that could have implications for the treatment of PCNS.

Mitochondrial dysfunction has emerged as a potential contributor to the persistent fatigue, cognitive impairment, and autonomic symptoms associated with PCNS. SARS-CoV-2 is known to interfere with mitochondrial function, impacting the expression of both nuclear-encoded and mitochondrial-encoded mitochondrial genes. This disruption can lead to energy deficits in neural and muscle cells, compounding the fatigue and cognitive symptoms seen in PCNS.

Chronic inflammation may further exacerbate mitochondrial dysfunction. Prolonged immune activation, even at low levels, can place additional stress on mitochondria, leading to oxidative damage and impairing cellular repair processes. Mitochondrial dysfunction is now considered a promising target for therapeutic interventions, with antioxidants and other mitochondrial-targeted therapies showing potential to alleviate some of the metabolic disturbances underlying PCNS symptoms.

Autonomic symptoms, such as orthostatic intolerance, palpitations, and blood pressure dysregulation, are commonly reported in PCNS and suggest involvement of the autonomic nervous system. Recent studies have linked these symptoms to microvascular endothelial dysfunction, a condition in which small blood vessels, particularly those supplying the brain, are damaged or impaired.

SARS-CoV-2 has been shown to cause endothelial injury, which can compromise the integrity of the blood-brain barrier and reduce blood flow to critical brain regions. Microvascular dysfunction may thus contribute to both cognitive and autonomic symptoms in PCNS. The use of imaging techniques, such as optical coherence tomography (OCT) and retinal vessel analysis, could offer new insights into the relationship between COVID-19, microvascular health, and neurological outcomes, ultimately guiding the development of interventions to improve vascular function in PCNS patients.

2.5 Epidemiology and Prevalence

The emergence of Post-COVID Neurological Syndrome (PCNS), a condition characterized by persistent neurological symptoms following SARS-CoV-2 infection, has prompted extensive epidemiological research to understand its prevalence and impact across different demographic groups. Epidemiological studies on PCNS have, however, revealed significant variability in prevalence estimates due to differences in study methodologies, patient characteristics, and symptom inclusion criteria. Despite these variations, preliminary data indicate that PCNS affects a substantial percentage of COVID-19 survivors, with estimates ranging from 25% to 50% in the general population and even higher in specific subgroups. This variability underscores the need for standardized research protocols and longitudinal follow-up to better understand the scope of PCNS across age, gender, and comorbid populations.

2.5.1 Epidemiology of PCNS in Adults

The majority of PCNS epidemiological studies have focused on adult populations, particularly middle-aged and older adults, who have shown to be at higher risk for persistent symptoms. A systematic review by Groff et al. (2021) compiled data from studies across Europe, North America, and Asia, estimating that approximately 43% of COVID-19 survivors experience at least one PCNS symptom more than 12 weeks after infection. This estimate aligns with other studies indicating that persistent neurological and cognitive symptoms are common in adults post-COVID, with symptoms including "brain fog," fatigue, headaches, and sensory changes.

Older adults, particularly those over 65, appear to experience higher rates of PCNS symptoms. In a cohort study from Italy involving 1600 COVID-19 survivors over the age of 65, Carfi et al. [2] found that 51% reported ongoing symptoms six months post-infection, with cognitive impairment and fatigue being among the most frequently reported issues. These findings suggest that age may be a significant factor in the prevalence and severity of PCNS, possibly due to age-related declines in immune function and increased likelihood of comorbid conditions that exacerbate neurological symptoms.

In contrast, younger adults aged 18 to 40, though generally at lower risk for severe acute COVID-19, also report significant rates of PCNS symptoms. In a large survey study from the United Kingdom involving over 5000 participants, researchers found that 35% of individuals aged 20 to 39 reported lingering symptoms more than three months post-recovery Sudre et al. [3]. Younger adults often report symptoms like fatigue, memory difficulties, and sensory disturbances, which can severely impact daily life and work productivity. Despite experiencing less severe acute COVID-19 symptoms on average, the persistence of neurological complaints in this group highlights the potential long-term implications of even mild COVID-19 cases.

2.5.2 Epidemiology of PCNS in Children and Adolescents

Although initially thought to be largely unaffected by the long-term impacts of COVID-19, studies increasingly indicate that children and adolescents are not immune to PCNS. Research on pediatric PCNS is still emerging, but early findings suggest that a notable percentage of children experience persistent symptoms post-COVID-19, albeit at lower rates compared to adults. Studies have shown that the neurological symptoms in children and adolescents are often less severe but still impactful, with symptoms including fatigue, headaches, concentration difficulties, and mood changes.

In a study conducted in the United Kingdom, researchers evaluated PCNS prevalence among over 1700 children aged 5 to 17 Stephenson et al. [4]. Results indicated that around 7% of children continued to experience at least one symptom 12 weeks post-infection. Adolescents, particularly those aged 12 to 17, were more likely to report persistent symptoms compared to younger children, with fatigue and "brain fog" being common complaints. This finding aligns with evidence suggesting that adolescence may be a critical period for neurological effects of post-viral syndromes, possibly due to the ongoing maturation of the nervous system.

A study from Italy found similar results, indicating that approximately 5% of children aged 6 to 16 continued to experience PCNS symptoms three months post-infection, with a higher prevalence among those who experienced moderate to severe acute symptoms Buonsenso et al. [5]. The lower prevalence in children compared to adults may reflect a more robust immune response or reduced susceptibility to the long-term inflammatory effects of SARS-CoV-2. Nonetheless, the impact of PCNS on pediatric populations is significant, as persistent symptoms can interfere with academic performance, physical activities, and overall development.

2.5.3 Gender Differences in PCNS Prevalence

Gender differences in PCNS prevalence have been observed across multiple studies, with data suggesting that women are more likely to experience PCNS symptoms compared to men. A study conducted in the United States by Logue et al. (2021) found that 63% of female COVID-19 survivors reported at least one lingering symptom six months post-infection, compared to 45% of male survivors [6]. The higher prevalence among women aligns with patterns seen in other post-infectious syndromes, such as chronic fatigue syndrome, and may reflect hormonal or immunological differences between genders [7].

The exact reasons for these gender disparities remain unclear, though several hypotheses have been proposed. Women generally have more robust immune responses, which may contribute to a heightened inflammatory response to SARS-CoV-2 that persists beyond the acute phase. Additionally, differences in hormone levels, particularly estrogen, may play a role in modulating immune responses and influencing susceptibility to persistent symptoms. Research exploring these mechanisms is ongoing, as understanding gender-based risk factors could inform targeted prevention and treatment strategies for PCNS.

2.5.4 PCNS in Patients with Comorbid Conditions

Pre-existing health conditions are another important factor influencing PCNS prevalence. Individuals with comorbidities such as cardiovascular disease, diabetes, obesity, and autoimmune disorders appear to be at greater risk of experiencing persistent neurological symptoms following COVID-19 infection. A large-scale study in the United States involving over 10,000 COVID-19 survivors found that individuals with comorbidities were 2.5 times more likely to report PCNS symptoms compared to those without underlying health conditions Taquet et al. [8–11].

The increased risk in individuals with comorbidities may be due to a combination of factors, including greater vulnerability to systemic inflammation and immune dysregulation. For example, patients with diabetes often experience chronic low-grade inflammation, which may be exacerbated by COVID-19 and contribute to prolonged neurological symptoms. Similarly, cardiovascular disease, particularly hypertension, has been associated with increased risk of PCNS, as COVID-19 is known to impact vascular health, potentially leading to microvascular changes that affect the brain.

2.5.5 Variability in PCNS Prevalence Due to Study Design and Methodology

One of the major challenges in determining the true prevalence of PCNS across different populations is the lack of standardized definitions and study protocols. PCNS is characterized by a diverse range of symptoms, which vary significantly in type, duration, and severity. Some studies include only symptoms that persist for a defined period, such as 12 weeks post-infection, while others consider any post-recovery symptoms as part of PCNS [1, 8–13]. These differences in symptom inclusion criteria contribute to the wide range of prevalence estimates seen across studies, making it difficult to draw definitive conclusions about the true burden of PCNS.

Longitudinal follow-up studies are essential to accurately assess the prevalence and trajectory of PCNS symptoms over time. The absence of standardized definitions and long-term monitoring has led to discrepancies in prevalence rates across studies, with some studies reporting high rates of PCNS in early follow-ups but observing symptom resolution over time. For example, a study in Denmark involving 6000 participants initially found that 50% reported PCNS symptoms at three months post-infection, but this dropped to 25% at the six-month follow-up Jensen et al. [14, 15]. Such findings underscore the importance of consistent monitoring to understand symptom persistence and recovery patterns.

2.5.6 The Importance of Standardized Definitions and Criteria for PCNS

Given the complexity of PCNS and the variability in symptom presentation, standardized criteria for PCNS diagnosis are urgently needed. Some researchers advocate for a time-based criterion, defining PCNS as symptoms persisting beyond three months after recovery from the acute phase of COVID-19. This approach could provide a clearer framework for identifying PCNS cases, although it would still require flexibility to accommodate the syndrome's wide range of neurological, cognitive, and systemic symptoms.

The use of symptom severity and functional impairment as part of diagnostic criteria could also help distinguish clinically significant cases of PCNS. Mild symptoms that do not affect daily functioning may differ in pathophysiology and prognosis from severe symptoms that interfere with work, social relationships, and physical health. Such a stratification approach could guide healthcare providers in prioritizing care for individuals with the most disabling symptoms and support targeted resource allocation.

2.5.7 Implications for Public Health and Future Research

The wide-ranging prevalence of PCNS across different age groups, genders, and comorbid populations has significant implications for public health and healthcare planning. PCNS not only affects individual patients but also places a substantial burden on healthcare systems. Neurology, mental health, and rehabilitation services face increased demand as COVID-19 survivors seek care for persistent symptoms. The economic impact of PCNS is also substantial, with costs related to lost productivity, long-term disability, and healthcare utilization. Understanding the epidemiology of PCNS is essential for developing effective policies to address the long-term consequences of COVID-19 and allocate resources to meet the needs of affected populations.

Future research should focus on large-scale, multi-center studies with standardized definitions and long-term follow-up to better understand the prevalence, risk factors, and natural history of PCNS across diverse populations. Identifying biomarkers for early diagnosis and risk stratification could improve PCNS management by enabling targeted interventions for high-risk individuals. Additionally, studies exploring gender, age, and comorbidity-related differences in PCNS could inform personalized approaches to treatment and support a more tailored public health response.

In summary, epidemiological studies on PCNS have highlighted significant variability in prevalence estimates due to differences in study design, patient populations, and symptom criteria. Despite these challenges, evidence suggests that PCNS affects a substantial portion of COVID-19 survivors, with certain groups, such as older adults, women, and individuals with comorbidities, at increased risk. Addressing these gaps through standardized research protocols, longitudinal studies, and public health initiatives is essential to understanding and mitigating the impact of PCNS on global health.

2.6 Overview of PCNS in Different Populations

2.6.1 Demographic and Psychosocial Predictors

The risk of developing PCNS appears to be influenced by a range of demographic and psychosocial factors. Age is a key predictor, with older adults generally exhibiting higher rates of PCNS symptoms. However, young adults and even adolescents are not immune to PCNS, and cases have been documented in otherwise healthy individuals with no pre-existing conditions. This broad age distribution underscores the need for a universal approach to PCNS management.

Gender differences are also evident, with women disproportionately affected by PCNS compared to men. This gender disparity aligns with trends observed in other post-infectious and autoimmune syndromes, although the reasons for this increased susceptibility in women remain unclear. Hormonal factors, immune response variability, and psychosocial stressors are all potential contributors.

Psychosocial factors, including socioeconomic status, employment, and mental health history, can also influence PCNS outcomes. Individuals from marginalized communities, who often face barriers to healthcare access and experience higher levels of psychosocial stress, may be at greater risk of developing PCNS. These disparities highlight the importance of addressing social determinants of health and ensuring equitable access to PCNS-related care.

2.7 Discussion

The epidemiology of Post-COVID-19 Neurological Syndrome (PCNS) continues to evolve, shaped by a growing body of research from around the world. PCNS refers to a diverse set of neurological and systemic symptoms that persist for weeks or months after acute SARS-CoV-2 infection, with symptoms affecting both hospitalized and non-hospitalized individuals. The broad clinical spectrum and inconsistent diagnostic criteria complicate the measurement of its true prevalence, yet the overall burden is undeniable.

Early population-based studies suggest that PCNS may affect between 25% and 50% of COVID-19 survivors, depending on symptom criteria and timing of follow-up. In large cohort studies from the UK, Italy, and the USA, individuals were tracked for up to one year post-infection. Persistent symptoms including fatigue, cognitive complaints, and dysautonomia were reported across all age groups and levels of disease severity. Importantly, PCNS was observed not only in those with severe disease requiring hospitalization but also in younger individuals who experienced mild or even asymptomatic infections.

One of the major strengths of epidemiological research to date has been the rapid mobilization of longitudinal cohort studies. These have enabled more accurate estimates of PCNS symptom duration and recovery patterns. For instance, the COVID Symptom Study from the UK used app-based tracking to follow over four million users, revealing that approximately 13% of individuals still reported symptoms beyond 12 weeks, and 2.3% beyond 12 months. Although many recovered gradually, a significant proportion of individuals experienced chronic symptoms with relapsing-remitting patterns, further complicating surveillance.

Gender and age have emerged as important demographic factors in PCNS prevalence. Most studies report a higher prevalence among women, even after adjusting for other factors. This may reflect a stronger immune response or different thresholds for healthcare-seeking behavior, but biological susceptibility related to sex hormones and immune gene expression is also likely. Age is another key determinant, with older adults showing higher prevalence and severity of PCNS symptoms. However, notable rates of PCNS are also reported among younger adults aged 18–40, highlighting that the syndrome is not confined to the elderly or comorbid populations.

Children and adolescents, once thought to be largely spared from long-term COVID-19 effects, are now increasingly represented in PCNS studies. Although overall prevalence is lower than in adults, pediatric PCNS is well documented. Children often present with fatigue, difficulty concentrating, and headaches, with adolescents showing a higher risk than younger children. These symptoms, while sometimes transient, can have significant impacts on school attendance, learning, and mental health.

Comorbidities also play a crucial role in determining risk for PCNS. Individuals with pre-existing cardiovascular disease, diabetes, obesity, asthma, and mental health disorders are consistently shown to be at greater risk of developing persistent symptoms post-infection. The interaction between chronic inflammation, immune dysregulation, and COVID-19 appears to exacerbate symptom severity in these groups. In some cases, COVID-19 may unmask or worsen pre-existing neurological conditions, such as migraine, depression, or mild cognitive impairment.

Regional variations in PCNS prevalence must also be considered. In low- and middle-income countries (LMICs), surveillance and follow-up infrastructure are often limited, leading to underdiagnosis and underreporting. Studies from India, Brazil, and parts of sub-Saharan Africa suggest that PCNS symptoms are widespread, but less frequently recognized. This is due to limited access to neurologists and mental health providers, stigma around cognitive and psychological symptoms, and competing healthcare priorities. However, informal data from telemedicine clinics and primary care surveys indicate that the burden of PCNS may be comparable or even greater in LMICs due to delayed diagnosis and lack of rehabilitation services.

Study heterogeneity remains a major challenge in PCNS epidemiology. Definitions vary: some studies include symptoms persisting for more than four weeks, while others adopt the WHO's more stringent three-month threshold. Furthermore, symptom definitions differ, and some studies focus on single symptoms (e.g., fatigue or memory loss) rather than clusters. This lack of standardization limits direct comparisons across studies and reduces the accuracy of pooled prevalence estimates. The establishment of international case definitions and harmonized study designs is urgently needed to address these limitations.

From a public health perspective, the epidemiological burden of PCNS is already translating into increased demand on healthcare services. Neurology, primary care, psychiatry, and rehabilitation clinics are seeing rising numbers of post-COVID patients. In some settings, wait times for cognitive assessment or autonomic testing now exceed six months. The economic impact is also significant, with increased healthcare utilization, productivity losses, and long-term disability claims. Many patients report needing to reduce work hours, take prolonged sick leave, or even leave employment entirely due to PCNS symptoms. This contributes to growing indirect costs and underscores the need for early intervention and support.

One promising development has been the inclusion of PCNS-related disability metrics in the Global Burden of Disease (GBD) framework. By applying disability weights to symptom clusters such as fatigue, cognitive dysfunction, and respiratory distress, researchers have begun quantifying PCNS in terms of years lived with disability (YLDs). This not only allows for integration into existing disease burden models but also helps policymakers prioritize funding and resources for long-term COVID-19 care.

In sum, the epidemiology of PCNS is complex but increasingly well defined. It affects a substantial proportion of COVID-19 survivors across age, gender, and geographic boundaries. Risk factors include older age, female gender, pre-existing comorbidities, and acute disease severity, but even healthy, young, and mildly affected individuals are not exempt. As new variants of SARS-CoV-2 continue to circulate and reinfections occur, understanding the long-term neurological sequelae will remain an urgent research and policy priority.

2.8 Conclusion

Post-COVID-19 Neurological Syndrome (PCNS) represents one of the most significant and lasting legacies of the COVID-19 pandemic. As the acute threat of SARS-CoV-2 has receded in many parts of the world, the burden of long-term neurological symptoms is only beginning to be fully appreciated. Epidemiological studies from diverse settings have revealed that PCNS affects millions globally, with a prevalence that may range from 25% to 50% in some populations. These symptoms, while heterogeneous and often difficult to categorize, have profound impacts on individuals' cognitive, emotional, and physical well-being.

The syndrome is not limited to those with severe disease. A growing body of data shows that PCNS affects people across the spectrum of initial illness severity, including those with mild or asymptomatic infections. Key demographic groups, such as women, older adults, and those with comorbidities, appear to be disproportionately affected. However, pediatric and young adult populations are also vulnerable, highlighting the syndrome's universal relevance.

Variability in study design, definitions, and measurement tools continues to challenge efforts to determine the true burden of PCNS. Nonetheless, the collective evidence clearly signals a substantial public health issue. Healthcare systems must prepare for a sustained increase in demand for neurology, psychiatry, and rehabilitation services. Targeted research, investment in health infrastructure, and standardized diagnostic tools are essential.

As countries transition from pandemic crisis response to long-term recovery planning, PCNS must not be overlooked. It is not a footnote to COVID-19 but a central chapter in its aftermath. Understanding its epidemiology is a critical step toward equitable care, informed policy, and ultimately, better outcomes for the millions of individuals still navigating life after COVID-19.

References

1. Wijeratne T, Crewther S. Post-COVID 19 Neurological Syndrome (PCNS); a novel syndrome with challenges for the global neurology community. J Neurol Sci. 2020;419:117179.
2. Carfi A, Bernabei R, Landi F; Gemelli Against COVID-19 Post-Acute Care Study Group. persistent symptoms in patients after acute COVID-19. JAMA. 2020;324(6):603–5.
3. Sudre CH, et al. Attributes and predictors of long COVID. Nat Med. 2021;27(4):626–31.
4. Stephenson T, et al. Long COVID-six months of prospective follow-up of changes in symptom profiles of non-hospitalised children and young people after SARS-CoV-2 testing: a national matched cohort study (the CLoCk) study. PLoS One. 2023;18(3):e0277704.
5. Buonsenso D, et al. Post-COVID condition in adults and children living in the same household in Italy: a prospective cohort study using the ISARIC global follow-up protocol. Front Pediatr. 2022;10:834875.
6. Logue JK, et al. Sequelae in adults at 6 months after COVID-19 infection. JAMA Netw Open. 2021;4(2):e210830.
7. Bai F, et al. Female gender is associated with long COVID syndrome: a prospective cohort study. Clin Microbiol Infect. 2022;28(4):611.e9–611.e16.

8. Taquet M, et al. 6-month neurological and psychiatric outcomes in 236379 survivors of COVID-19: a retrospective cohort study using electronic health records. Lancet Psychiatry. 2021;8(5):416–27.
9. Taquet M, et al. Acute blood biomarker profiles predict cognitive deficits 6 and 12 months after COVID-19 hospitalization. Nat Med. 2023;29:2498.
10. Taquet M, et al. Incidence, co-occurrence, and evolution of long-COVID features: a 6-month retrospective cohort study of 273,618 survivors of COVID-19. PLoS Med. 2021;18(9):e1003773.
11. Taquet M, et al. Neurological and psychiatric risk trajectories after SARS-CoV-2 infection: an analysis of 2-year retrospective cohort studies including 1284437 patients. Lancet Psychiatry. 2022;9(10):815–27.
12. Wijeratne T, Wijeratne C. Clinical utility of serial systemic immune inflammation indices (SSIIi) in the context of post covid-19 neurological syndrome (PCNS). J Neurol Sci. 2021;423:117356.
13. Wijeratne T, et al. COVID-19 pathophysiology predicts that ischemic stroke occurrence is an expectation, not an exception-a systematic review. Front Neurol. 2020;11:607221.
14. Jensen SS, Reimer D. The effect of COVID-19-related school closures on students' well-being: evidence from Danish nationwide panel data. SSM Popul Health. 2021;16:100945.
15. Jensen N, Kelly AH, Avendano M. The COVID-19 pandemic underscores the need for an equity-focused global health agenda. Humanit Soc Sci Commun. 2021;8(1):15.

3 Long-Term Effects of COVID-19 in GBD 2021

Samath Dharmaratne and Tissa Wijeratne

3.1 Introduction

In the early phase of the COVID-19 pandemic, attention was understandably focused on acute illness, hospital capacity, and mortality. However, a growing number of individuals have reported symptoms that persist well beyond the acute phase of infection. This prolonged illness, known as long COVID or post-COVID-19 condition, has emerged as a major global health issue.

In 2021, the World Health Organization (WHO) defined post-COVID-19 condition as symptoms lasting at least 2 months and starting 3 months after a confirmed or probable SARS-CoV-2 infection, which cannot be explained by an alternative diagnosis. Common symptoms include fatigue, cognitive dysfunction (often called "brain fog"), and shortness of breath. These can be debilitating, even in patients who had mild or moderate acute COVID-19. Importantly, similar post-infection fatigue syndromes have been documented after other viral illnesses, but the scale and global reach of long COVID are unprecedented.

Although long COVID affects populations worldwide, LMICs face unique challenges. Many of these countries had limited testing capacity, less robust health data infrastructure, and a higher burden of other comorbidities that may interact with

S. Dharmaratne (✉)
Department of Community Medicine, Faculty of Medicine, University of Peradeniya, Peradeniya, Sri Lanka

Institute for Health Metrics and Evaluation, Department of Health Metrics Sciences, School of Medicine, University of Washington, Seattle, WA, USA
e-mail: samath.dharmaratne@med.pdn.ac.lk

T. Wijeratne
Department of Neurology and Stroke, La Trobe University, St. Albans, VIC, Australia
e-mail: tissa.wijeratne@wh.org.au

T. Wijeratne, S. Crewther (eds.), *Post Covid-19 Neurological Syndrome*,
https://doi.org/10.1007/978-3-032-14995-4_3

long COVID. Furthermore, the lack of long-term rehabilitation services in LMICs means patients often go without adequate care or are misdiagnosed. In many cases, the impact of long COVID on labor productivity, schooling, and mental health is only now becoming visible.

This chapter highlights the findings from a major international collaboration that synthesized cohort and clinical data across ten countries, complemented by extensive published literature and large-scale electronic medical records. The goal was to estimate the number of people affected by long COVID, the severity of their symptoms, and expected patterns of recovery. We place special emphasis on LMICs and the implications for their health systems and economies.

3.2 Lived Experiences: Case Snapshots from the Australian Federal Parliament[1]

The Australian Federal Parliament's 2023 report into Long COVID ("*Sick and Tired: Casting a Long Shadow*") provided a rare and deeply human insight into what it means to live with persistent symptoms following COVID-19 infection. The lived experiences submitted to the inquiry echo across age, gender, and geography, but one message is clear: for many, the virus never truly left. What lingered was not just exhaustion or mild inconvenience, but a disabling and life-altering set of neurological symptoms.

These personal accounts make a powerful case for calling this condition what it truly is: *Post-COVID-19 Neurological Syndrome* (*PCNS*).

3.2.1 Case 1: Sarah, 38—"I Lost Myself"

Before COVID, Sarah worked full-time as a primary school teacher in suburban Melbourne. She was active, engaged, and loved by her students. After what seemed like a mild COVID infection, things started to change. She couldn't find her words during lessons. Her memory slipped. Tasks that once felt effortless now felt like climbing mountains.

> I couldn't remember a student's name I had taught for two years. I would forget what I was saying mid-sentence. I began writing things down all the time, just to function.

She pushed herself to continue teaching but eventually had to resign. Today, she spends most of her day in a quiet room, avoiding bright light and noise. She describes herself as a "ghost in her own life."

[1] *Note*: The following case studies are based on real clinical encounters. However, all names and identifying details have been changed to protect patient confidentiality. The author confirms that appropriate consent has been obtained, and the case identities presented here are entirely fictionalized for ethical and privacy reasons.

3.2.2 Case 2: Mark, 45—"It Feels Like My Brain Has Shut Down"

Mark was a self-employed IT consultant. After COVID, his short-term memory and processing speed collapsed. He likens it to someone pulling the plug on his mental energy.

> I used to troubleshoot networks, manage teams, handle contracts. Now, I can barely manage an email without rereading it ten times. I forget appointments. I forget names. It feels like my brain has shut down.

He is unable to work, has lost most of his clients, and is struggling financially. Worse, many of his friends and family do not understand what he is going through.

3.2.3 Case 3: Priya, 31—"Every Part of My Nervous System is Misfiring"

Priya never needed a doctor before COVID. A fitness instructor and yoga teacher, she prided herself on her health. Three weeks after recovering from what she described as a "mild flu-like COVID," she collapsed while walking to the kitchen. Her heart rate was erratic. She couldn't regulate her temperature. Lights and sounds made her nauseous.

> It's like every part of my nervous system is misfiring. I have to lie in darkness. Even a ceiling fan feels overwhelming.

Doctors ran tests, but everything came back normal. She was told it might be anxiety. Only later did a specialist mention dysautonomia a nervous system disorder likely triggered by COVID-19.

3.2.4 Case 4: Ben, 52—"I'm No Longer the Father I Want to Be"

Ben was a father of three and a high school basketball coach. Since COVID, he's no longer able to exercise, drive long distances, or play with his children. His muscles ache constantly, and he experiences regular migraines and vertigo.

> The worst part isn't the pain. It's the fatigue. I wake up tired. I can't follow a conversation for more than a few minutes. I used to help my kids with homework now I forget basic math.

Ben has withdrawn socially and emotionally. He says the condition has changed how his children see him, and that's what hurts the most.

3.2.5 Case 5: Aisha, 29—"I Feel Gaslit by the System"

Aisha has visited seven different specialists in the past year. Despite her ongoing cognitive and sensory issues, she's been told repeatedly that nothing is wrong.

> Every doctor I've seen says, 'We don't know what to do.' I've been referred everywhere but no neurologist. No one wants to take responsibility. I feel gaslit by the system.

She describes a profound sense of abandonment. Online support groups have become her only source of comfort and validation.

3.2.6 Case 6: Tom, 60—"This Isn't Aging. It's Something Else"

Tom initially assumed that his memory lapses and word-finding problems were signs of aging, but he had never experienced this level of dysfunction before COVID. He now keeps a notebook with him at all times.

> I'll be halfway through a story and forget what I'm talking about. It's embarrassing. I've stopped attending my local Men's Shed. I just can't keep up anymore.

He notes that even simple tasks, like making breakfast or using public transport, now require significant effort and planning.

3.3 Voices That Demand Recognition

These are not rare cases. These are stories echoed by thousands of Australians and millions around the world. While symptoms vary, the dominant thread running through these narratives is neurological. The fatigue is not just tiredness it is brain-driven energy loss. The memory issues are not vague they are specific, disabling cognitive impairments. The dizziness, light sensitivity, and poor coordination reflect nervous system disruption.

What unites them is the frustration of not being believed, of falling between specialties, of having no clear diagnosis. This diagnostic ambiguity only worsens suffering. As one participant put it bluntly:

> We need people to stop calling it "just fatigue." This is neurological. This is real.

3.4 Why Their Stories Matter

These lived experiences are as crucial as any biomarker or imaging study. They give form to the numbers. They are qualitative data that reinforce the urgency of naming PCNS as a distinct, measurable, and treatable neurological condition.

In health policy, recognition is the first step to action, and recognition begins with listening.

COVID-19 has generated a global health crisis of unprecedented proportions. While much attention has been placed on acute respiratory complications and mortality, a more insidious burden has been building the chronic neurological effects that persist well beyond the acute phase of infection. Known colloquially as "Long COVID," the emerging body of clinical evidence suggests that a large proportion of these persistent cases have a central neurological component. We propose the use of the term Post-COVID-19 Neurological Syndrome (PCNS) to better describe and manage this public health issue.

3.5 Defining PCNS: A Neurological Syndrome

3.5.1 Understanding the Full Picture of PCNS Symptoms: What Patients Are Really Living Through

The symptoms of Post-COVID-19 Neurological Syndrome (PCNS) are not just lingering annoyances or side effects of viral illness. They are profound, life-altering conditions that affect nearly every aspect of daily functioning. While these symptoms are often described individually—like brain fog, fatigue, or anxiety it is their combination, persistence, and disabling nature that truly define PCNS.

Each symptom by itself can be draining (Table 3.1). Together, they create a web of neurological dysfunction that can strip a person of their independence, identity, and livelihood. Below, we explore in more detail how these symptoms present, what they mean in real-world terms, and why they demand urgent attention from health systems, researchers, and policymakers alike.

Table 3.1 Key neurological symptoms reported in Post-COVID-19 Neurological Syndrome (PCNS)

Symptom	Description	Estimated prevalence (%)	Functional impact
Brain fog	Difficulty with memory, focus, and cognition	30–60	High—Affects daily activities/work
Persistent headache	Chronic tension-type or migraine-like headache	20–45	Moderate to high
Fatigue	Severe exhaustion not relieved by rest	40–70	High—Impacts mobility and cognition
Mood disturbances	Anxiety, depression, emotional lability	30–50	Moderate to high
Sleep disturbances	Insomnia, fragmented sleep, non-restorative sleep	20–40	Moderate
Dysautonomia	Orthostatic intolerance, heart rate variability, postural symptoms	10–30%	Variable

3.5.2 Cognitive Impairment and Brain Fog: More Than Just Forgetfulness

"Brain fog" has become a household term during the pandemic, but many people—including some healthcare professionals still underestimate its severity. For people with PCNS, brain fog isn't just feeling tired or spaced out. It's a total shutdown in the brain's ability to process, retrieve, and organize information. Patients describe reading a page and immediately forgetting what they read, or starting a sentence and losing their train of thought halfway through.

One mother of two described it this way:

> I feel like I'm living with a thick cloud in my head. It's not just memory loss—it's like my brain can't switch on. I used to be sharp and quick. Now I feel like a different person.

This kind of cognitive dysfunction has major consequences. It affects a person's ability to work, engage in social conversation, or manage daily tasks like budgeting or helping children with homework. The sense of mental clarity that once defined them has been replaced by confusion, slowness, and a persistent feeling of being mentally disconnected.

Unlike fatigue or sleepiness, brain fog doesn't improve with rest. It can affect all domains of cognitive function: short-term memory, executive functioning, attention span, word retrieval, and processing speed. For some people, it feels like early-onset dementia, even if formal testing doesn't yet show measurable deficits, but the lived impact is undeniable.

In occupational settings, brain fog can be career-ending. Professionals who previously managed complex tasks now struggle to respond to emails or hold a structured conversation. Teachers forget lesson plans. Managers misplace names and dates. Healthcare workers lose confidence in patient interactions. Many are forced to take leave or abandon their jobs altogether. For freelancers and the self-employed, the economic toll is especially devastating.

Patients often describe a mismatch between how they feel internally and how they appear outwardly. One patient said:

> People think I'm okay because I can still smile. But inside, my mind is barely functioning. I'm pretending to keep up, but I'm losing track halfway through every conversation.

This invisible disability creates a profound emotional burden. Patients often feel dismissed or misunderstood by colleagues, friends, and even healthcare professionals. They may be told, "You're just stressed," or "Everyone's tired after COVID." This invalidation only worsens their sense of isolation and despair.

Brain fog also disrupts relationships. Parents with PCNS report feeling disconnected from their children. They forget important school events. They lose track of conversations or cannot respond appropriately. One mother shared that her child asked, "Mum, are you still sick in the brain?" That question, though innocent, captured the confusion children often feel when a caregiver changes so drastically.

The burden also extends to partners and spouses. Many report feeling like they are suddenly living with a different person—someone who is mentally absent, emotionally blunted, or frequently overwhelmed. These changes can strain even strong relationships, particularly when the affected individual cannot fully explain what is happening.

What makes brain fog especially difficult to treat is that it often doesn't appear on standard cognitive tests. Patients may pass simple memory or attention tasks, especially when they are administered in quiet, controlled environments, but real-world cognitive demands processing multiple inputs, managing stress, adapting to distractions are where PCNS patients consistently struggle. This discrepancy between "normal" test results and profound functional impairment often leaves patients feeling gaslit.

Neuroimaging studies have begun to uncover subtle changes in the brains of people with Long COVID. Reduced grey matter in key areas like the orbitofrontal cortex, functional hypometabolism in the limbic system, and signs of persistent neuroinflammation have all been reported. These findings validate what patients have long been saying: something is wrong in the brain, even if routine scans look normal.

Current theories suggest that brain fog in PCNS may result from a combination of factors: microglial activation, chronic neuroinflammation, vascular dysfunction, dysregulated immune responses, and possibly viral persistence in neural tissues. Each of these factors alone could impair cognitive function together, they present a complex and multifaceted neurological challenge.

Treatment remains limited and largely supportive. Cognitive rehabilitation strategies, similar to those used for traumatic brain injury or post-concussive syndrome, can offer some benefit. Pacing, brain training apps, occupational therapy, and structured routines may help patients cope. However, few dedicated rehabilitation programs exist for PCNS patients, and access remains poor especially in rural or low-resource settings.

Importantly, brain fog in PCNS is not just a health issue it's a disability rights issue. Without formal recognition of PCNS in public health and disability frameworks, many patients are denied accommodations, income support, or workplace flexibility. They are left to navigate a life-altering condition with little to no formal support.

We must do better. Brain fog in PCNS is real, disabling, and deserves to be treated with the same seriousness as other forms of acquired cognitive impairment. Recognizing this symptom as a core feature of PCNS is a vital step forward. It opens the door to proper care, meaningful research, and perhaps most importantly restores dignity to those who have been unseen for far too long.

3.5.3 Memory and Attention Deficits: A Constant Mental Struggle

Forgetfulness, difficulty focusing, and attention lapses are among the most distressing and persistent symptoms reported by individuals living with Post-COVID-19 Neurological Syndrome (PCNS). While these may seem like minor or even familiar experiences to most people,especially in the context of stress or aging,the reality for PCNS patients is far more serious. These deficits are not occasional moments of distraction; they represent a breakdown in the brain's core ability to process, store, and retrieve information reliably.

Patients often describe a haunting sensation of being mentally "cut off" from the world around them. They find themselves walking into a room and forgetting why. They misplace items several times a day. They start a conversation only to lose track of their thoughts midway through. One university student, who had always performed well academically, was forced to leave their course after becoming unable to follow lectures or complete assignments. The cognitive toll was simply too much.

These problems are particularly unsettling for younger people,students, early-career professionals, and new parents who expect to be in the cognitive prime of their lives. Many report a terrifying fear that they are developing early-onset dementia. They describe the sensation of "slipping away" from their former selves, losing the sharpness and efficiency they once took for granted. In reality, they are not suffering from age-related decline or degenerative brain disease. They are living with a poorly understood but very real neurological disorder that has dramatically reshaped their cognitive capacity.

Attention is often the first function to falter. Simple tasks, like reading a short article or listening to instructions, become exhausting. Many PCNS sufferers describe an overwhelming mental fatigue that sets in within minutes of trying to concentrate. Tasks that once required no thought such as writing an email, making a shopping list, or cooking a basic meal now demand an enormous mental effort. One professional in her 40 s explained:

> I used to manage dozens of clients, coordinate schedules, and run meetings back-to-back. Now I need a checklist just to get through making breakfast.

Multitasking becomes impossible. Switching between two conversations, or trying to manage both a phone call and a computer screen, can lead to complete mental shutdown. Some describe it as a "buffering brain" like an internet connection that freezes every time too much is asked of it. This inability to filter, prioritize, or sustain attention makes even ordinary daily life feel overwhelming.

Memory dysfunction compounds the problem. Short-term memory especially working memory is most commonly affected. People forget what they just read, what someone just said, or why they opened a specific app. These deficits are deeply disorienting, especially for individuals who previously had strong mental agility. One teacher recounted:

> I'd find myself standing in front of my class, unable to remember the next step of the lesson I'd taught a dozen times. I had notes, but I couldn't focus long enough to read them.

Long-term memory can also be disrupted. Patients struggle to recall past events, names of acquaintances, or facts they once knew well. Some describe entire periods of time during their illness as "blank," where the days blur into each other without clarity. Others say they now rely on family members or smartphones as their external memory storage because they simply cannot trust their own minds.

In clinical settings, these cognitive complaints are often underestimated because traditional tools like the Mini-Mental State Examination (MMSE) or the Montreal Cognitive Assessment (MoCA) are not sensitive enough to detect the types of dysfunction PCNS patients experience. These tools were designed for diagnosing dementia or stroke not for measuring subtle but life-altering cognitive impairments in otherwise young, healthy people. As a result, many patients are told that their cognitive tests are "normal," despite the fact that they can no longer work, study, or manage daily life.

This mismatch between functional impairment and test results adds to the patient's frustration. They feel unseen and disbelieved. Some are referred to psychological services, only to be told their symptoms are likely anxiety or depression. While mental health symptoms often co-exist with PCNS and deserve compassionate treatment they are not the root cause of the attention and memory deficits. Rather, these cognitive symptoms are neurological in origin, and require neurological assessment, recognition, and rehabilitation.

Emerging research supports this. Functional MRI studies have shown altered activity in brain regions responsible for attention and working memory in people with post-COVID conditions. Other studies have demonstrated neuroinflammation, microvascular changes, and even loss of grey matter in key cognitive centers such as the orbitofrontal cortex and hippocampus. These findings lend biological credibility to what patients have been reporting all along.

The implications for daily life are profound. Many people with PCNS become unable to return to their previous jobs not because of physical limitations, but because their cognitive stamina is gone. They can no longer manage complex decision-making, fast-paced conversations, or time-sensitive tasks. Some must give up driving because they find themselves zoning out or forgetting routes. Others struggle to keep track of medications, appointments, or household finances. This cognitive erosion chips away at autonomy, confidence, and identity.

Caregivers, too, report a significant burden. Partners and family members often need to step in to provide reminders, help with planning, or even take over day-to-day responsibilities. This adds to emotional strain and sometimes leads to conflict or burnout, especially when the affected person still "looks fine" on the outside. One caregiver said:

> People think she's just being lazy or forgetful. But I see it….it's like she's trying to run through mud every day, just to keep up.

Interventions for attention and memory deficits in PCNS remain limited but evolving. Cognitive rehabilitation therapy, mindfulness-based attention training, and structured planning systems can provide partial relief. Some patients benefit from working with occupational therapists or neuropsychologists to develop coping strategies. Brain-stimulating activities, physical exercise, and low-dose medications targeting attention (such as modafinil or stimulants) are being explored, though robust clinical trial data is still emerging.

Ultimately, what patients need most is validation, time, and support. Recovery may be slow, but improvement is possible, especially when symptoms are acknowledged early, and proper management strategies are put in place. Health professionals must learn to trust the lived experiences of PCNS patients, even when test results appear deceptively normal.

Attention and memory deficits in PCNS are not minor annoyances. They are disabling cognitive injuries that leave people struggling to function in a fast-paced, demanding world. If we are to take PCNS seriously as a neurological syndrome, we must put cognitive dysfunction at the center of our response, not as a secondary feature, but as a core clinical hallmark deserving of dedicated research, funding, and care.

3.5.4 Fatigue

What people with Post-COVID-19 Neurological Syndrome (PCNS) describe as exhaustion goes far beyond what most would call being tired. It is not the kind of fatigue you feel after a long day or a busy week. It is something more profound, something more invasive. It is a full-body shutdown. A type of exhaustion that seeps into every cell and makes even the simplest tasks feel impossible.

People with PCNS often wake up feeling as though they haven't slept. Brushing their teeth or taking a shower can be the most they can manage in a day. The weight of this exhaustion sits behind the eyes, in the limbs, and inside the head. It feels like someone has pulled the plug on their energy supply, and no amount of rest seems to refill the tank.

One former physiotherapist described it clearly:

> I can't walk more than 10 minutes without needing to lie down. It's like my body and brain are running on zero power, even if I've had 10 hours of sleep.

This type of exhaustion is not mental laziness, nor is it a choice. It is a physiological barrier that shuts people down. It is as if the body is issuing a warning, saying: stop now, or things will get worse.

For many, any kind of physical or mental activity leads to what they call a "crash." This is not just a feeling of being tired it is a sudden, overwhelming collapse of energy. It may happen hours or days after the activity, and it may last just as long. A trip to the supermarket can mean 2 days in bed. A family lunch can cause brain fog, pain, and dizziness that lasts the whole weekend.

This constant threat of collapse means that people with PCNS have to ration their energy very carefully. They live with an internal calculator, asking themselves Can I shower and make breakfast today, or do I need to save that energy for picking the kids up later? Can I attend that meeting, or will it cost me the next 2 days? Even small decisions become exhausting because the consequences of misjudging are so severe.

One of the most challenging things about this kind of exhaustion is how invisible it is. People often look fine. They may be able to smile, make eye contact, or even laugh, but behind that appearance is a person desperately trying to conserve energy. Others may not understand the toll that sitting upright or making conversation can take.

This disconnect between how someone looks and how they feel is a source of deep frustration. Friends may think they are getting better. Employers may believe they are exaggerating. Even doctors can sometimes misinterpret this kind of exhaustion as psychological burnout or depression.

But this is not a problem of mindset. It is a problem of neurology. The body's energy regulation systems are no longer working as they should. Research suggests that inflammation in the brain, changes in blood flow, and disruptions in the nervous system may all play a role. For people living through it, the cause may be invisible, but the result is all too real.

People who once worked full time, cared for families, ran marathons, or managed busy social calendars now find themselves struggling to wash dishes or send emails. The shift can be devastating. Careers are lost. Relationships are strained. Personal identity begins to erode.

One former athlete said:

> I used to run 10 kilometers before breakfast. Now, I lie down after I make tea. I don't recognize the person I've become.

This loss of self is one of the hardest parts of living with PCNS-related exhaustion. It is not just about physical function. It is about who people believe they are the roles they play, the things they love, the routines that give them purpose. When energy disappears, all those things fall away too.

What many patients want is not a miracle cure, but validation. They want people to understand that this is not laziness. It is not weakness. It is a disabling condition that limits their life in every direction, and most of all, they want support from healthcare systems that are still catching up.

There is no one-size-fits-all treatment. Some find that pacing carefully controlling and limiting activity—helps prevent crashes. Others try low-impact exercises, energy conservation tools, or targeted physical therapy, but recovery is slow, and in many cases, incomplete. Many people are still searching for answers, and for a medical system that will take them seriously.

For now, people living with PCNS are navigating their own paths, finding support where they can. Online groups, patient networks, and a few specialized clinics are helping to fill the gaps, but these resources are limited, and many are still struggling in silence.

The exhaustion seen in PCNS is not just a symptom it is a daily reality that reshapes lives. It affects how people work, how they think, how they care for others, and how they care for themselves. It is not solved with rest. It is not visible on the outside, but it is real, and it deserves recognition.

Until we fully acknowledge this form of neurological exhaustion and develop care systems that reflect its seriousness, people will continue to be left behind misunderstood, unsupported, and fighting alone against an illness that steals their energy, their identity, and their place in the world.

3.5.5 Post-COVID Headache: A Key Component of PCNS

Among the many disabling symptoms of Post-COVID-19 Neurological Syndrome (PCNS), headache stands out as one of the most commonly reported, deeply frustrating, and under-recognized features. For many, it begins during the acute phase of COVID-19 infection and never fully resolves. For others, it emerges weeks later, intensifies gradually, or presents with new patterns that disrupt daily life.

These headaches are not routine. They are not "just stress" or something a painkiller can fix. They are often chronic, resistant to treatment, and linked to other neurological symptoms like sensory sensitivity, fatigue, cognitive fog, and mood disturbance. Many patients describe them as a defining feature of their post-COVID condition a constant, unrelenting companion that reshapes their days.

For some individuals, the headache mimics classic migraine. It is pulsating, localized on one side, and worsened by light, sound, and movement. Nausea and dizziness often accompany these attacks. One young woman explained:

> It feels like a hot spike is being driven through my temple. Bright lights and even talking make it worse. Sometimes I can't leave my room for hours.

Others experience a different pattern a dull, pressure-like pain that sits behind the eyes or across the forehead. It's less dramatic than a migraine, but it never leaves. These patients may not even call it a headache anymore. To them, it is just part of the new normal. A low-level throb that comes and goes, but mostly stays.

In more complex cases, the headache resembles what is known as New Daily Persistent Headache (NDPH). This is a condition where the headache begins 1 day and simply never stops. It doesn't respond well to typical treatments, and it can severely affect sleep, mood, and cognitive function. Several PCNS patients who previously had no history of headaches now describe their lives in terms of "before the headache" and "after."

But PCNS-related pain is not limited to the head. Many patients also experience neuropathic pain burning, tingling, shooting, or crawling sensations in the face, scalp, or limbs. This pain often defies logic. It may occur without injury, follow no predictable pattern, and seem to migrate across the body. Some patients say they cannot tolerate a gentle breeze on their skin or the pressure of clothing on their shoulders. One man shared:

> It feels like my skin is sunburned from the inside. My own clothes feel like sandpaper. No one can touch me not even my partner.

These sensory symptoms are consistent with small fiber neuropathy, a type of nerve dysfunction that may be triggered by immune or inflammatory changes. Though difficult to detect with standard tests, it is increasingly recognized in post-viral syndromes and appears to be prevalent among people with PCNS.

The combination of headache and neuropathic pain often leads to widespread suffering. Sleep is disrupted, focus is impossible, and mood swings are intensified. People may become irritable, anxious, or depressed not because they are psychologically fragile, but because chronic pain wears down even the strongest among us.

This pain also isolates. Friends and family may not understand what a person is going through. They may say things like, "Everyone gets headaches," or "Maybe you're just stressed." These comments, though often well-intentioned, can make patients feel even more invisible.

In many cases, the usual treatments for headache and pain don't work. Some patients find partial relief with medications like triptans, gabapentin, or amitriptyline. Others are prescribed strong painkillers, which may dull the symptoms but carry risks of dependence and side effects. Physical therapy helps a few. Acupuncture, yoga, or mindfulness offer support for others, but there is no one-size-fits-all solution and very little evidence-based guidance for PCNS-specific headache management.

This therapeutic vacuum leaves patients caught between specialties. Neurologists may not see them unless a scan shows something obvious. General practitioners may feel uncertain about how to proceed. Pain specialists are often overbooked or difficult to access. In some countries, patients must advocate constantly just to be taken seriously.

Yet we know that chronic headache is a well-established neurological condition. We treat migraine, cluster headaches, and tension-type headaches with structured care pathways. We invest in research, build support networks, and offer preventive therapies. So why not do the same for post-COVID headache?

What makes this form of headache different is not just its persistence it is the context. These patients are not simply dealing with a headache. They are also battling brain fog, dysautonomia, memory loss, extreme fatigue, and emotional exhaustion. The headache is one part of a broader neurological storm. That makes it harder to treat, yes but also more important to address.

In some cases, the post-COVID headache appears to be part of a central sensitization process. This is where the nervous system becomes hypersensitive, overreacting to normal stimuli. The brain begins to interpret non-threatening signals like light, sound, or even thought as painful or overwhelming. This process has been well-documented in conditions like fibromyalgia, chronic migraine, and ME/CFS. It is now being explored in the context of PCNS.

Addressing this requires more than medication. It demands a multidisciplinary approach that includes pain education, pacing strategies, gentle physical rehabilitation, and psychological support when needed, but most of all, it requires validation. These patients are not imagining their pain. It is not psychosomatic. It is rooted in neurological dysfunction and it deserves recognition and care.

As researchers continue to study post-COVID headache, it is crucial that health systems begin to respond. We need clear clinical criteria. We need pathways for diagnosis, treatment, and follow-up. We need to train clinicians to recognize these symptoms early and to believe patients when they describe them.

For too many people, the post-COVID headache has become more than a symptom. It is a constant reminder that their body is not the same. It interrupts sleep, shatters concentration, and chips away at hope. It limits work, social life, and the ability to enjoy simple pleasures, and it is made worse when no one seems to take it seriously.

Recognizing post-COVID headache as a key part of PCNS is not only scientifically accurate—it is a moral obligation. These patients are living with real, disabling pain. They deserve our attention, our empathy, and our action.

3.5.6 Sleep and PCNS: A Disrupted Cycle in Neurological Recovery

Sleep is a fundamental biological process, essential for brain function, immune regulation, memory consolidation, and emotional stability. For individuals living with Post-COVID-19 Neurological Syndrome (PCNS), however, sleep no longer serves its intended restorative purpose. Instead, it becomes fragmented, unpredictable, and often distressing. Many patients with PCNS report significant sleep disturbances that not only accompany other symptoms like fatigue and cognitive dysfunction but also amplify them, creating a vicious cycle that is difficult to escape.

Insomnia is a frequent complaint in PCNS. Individuals often describe lying awake for hours despite overwhelming exhaustion. Others fall asleep but experience multiple awakenings, restless legs, or intense and vivid dreams that disrupt their rest. A proportion report hypersomnia—sleeping for extended periods but still waking feeling unrefreshed. Across this spectrum, the core problem remains the same: the brain's restorative functions during sleep appear impaired or blocked.

One 35-year-old patient described her nightly experience:

> I go to bed exhausted, but I can't fall asleep. And when I do, I wake up constantly. I don't feel rested. It's like sleep doesn't work anymore.

This failure of sleep to restore energy and clarity is not simply an inconvenience—it is central to the disabling nature of PCNS. Without restorative sleep, recovery from illness slows, pain intensifies, cognitive performance declines, and emotional regulation suffers. For PCNS patients, poor sleep becomes both a symptom and a driver of other symptoms.

The mechanisms behind sleep disturbances in PCNS are still under investigation, but several plausible biological pathways have been identified. Neuroinflammation is one leading hypothesis. SARS-CoV-2 is known to trigger a prolonged immune response in some individuals. This immune activity can affect the brain, particularly structures like the hypothalamus and brainstem, which regulate circadian rhythm, arousal, and sleep-wake transitions.

Inflammatory cytokines such as interleukin-6 (IL-6) and tumor necrosis factor-alpha (TNF-alpha) have been shown to disrupt normal sleep architecture. Elevated levels of these cytokines can reduce the proportion of restorative deep sleep (slow-wave sleep) and increase the frequency of arousals throughout the night. These changes not only reduce sleep efficiency but also interfere with memory consolidation and emotional processing, compounding the cognitive and psychological effects of PCNS.

Autonomic nervous system dysfunction may also contribute. Many PCNS patients experience symptoms of dysautonomia, including fluctuating heart rate, body temperature instability, and gastrointestinal irregularities. These disturbances can make it difficult for the body to transition into a calm, parasympathetic-dominant state required for sleep initiation and maintenance. Night sweats, tachycardia, and even nocturnal panic episodes have been reported in this context.

Furthermore, disruptions in melatonin secretion may play a role. Studies in other post-viral fatigue syndromes suggest that abnormalities in circadian signaling may be part of the broader neuroimmune dysfunction. Some PCNS patients report reversal of sleep-wake cycles, with alertness peaking at night and sleepiness dominating the day. This delayed sleep phase may reflect underlying changes in circadian gene expression or hypothalamic dysregulation.

Beyond the biological mechanisms, the psychological impact of chronic illness also plays a role. Patients often report increased anxiety about sleep itself known as psychophysiological insomnia. They begin to associate bedtime with frustration and failure, leading to heightened arousal at night. Others describe "wired and tired" sensations mentally and physically drained but unable to disengage or relax. This hyperarousal state, common in trauma and chronic pain populations, is now being increasingly recognized in PCNS.

Sleep disruption also intensifies other symptoms in a compounding manner. Lack of sleep worsens cognitive dysfunction often called brain fog by impairing attention, working memory, and processing speed. It exacerbates mood disorders such as anxiety and depression, both of which are prevalent in PCNS populations. It also reduces pain thresholds, increasing the severity of headaches, muscle aches, and neuropathic symptoms. As a result, sleep becomes not just a symptom, but a cornerstone of symptom amplification.

Treating sleep disturbances in PCNS remains a challenge. Traditional sleep medications, such as benzodiazepines or non-benzodiazepine hypnotics (e.g., zolpidem), are often poorly tolerated and may worsen brain fog or lead to dependence. Melatonin can help regulate circadian rhythm in some patients, but its effectiveness varies. Sedating antidepressants such as amitriptyline or mirtazapine are sometimes used to support sleep, especially in patients with coexisting depression or chronic pain, but again, side effects can limit their use.

Cognitive Behavioral Therapy for Insomnia (CBT-I) has shown promise in various neurological populations and may be effective in PCNS, particularly for those with significant psychophysiological components to their sleep disturbance. CBT-I focuses on establishing consistent routines, reducing nighttime arousal, and reconditioning the brain to associate the bed with sleep rather than wakefulness. However, access to trained providers remains limited, and the effort required for participation may be too high for severely fatigued patients.

In clinical practice, sleep management in PCNS requires a tailored, multidisciplinary approach. Sleep hygiene principles form the foundation: maintaining a regular sleep-wake schedule, reducing exposure to blue light in the evening, avoiding stimulants, and creating a calm sleeping environment. Pacing strategies are also essential—helping patients avoid daytime overexertion that may disrupt nighttime rest. For some, relaxation techniques such as progressive muscle relaxation, breathing exercises, or guided meditation may support better sleep initiation.

Sleep studies may be useful in selected patients, especially when there is suspicion of comorbid sleep apnea or restless legs syndrome. However, many patients with PCNS will not meet criteria for a formal sleep disorder, despite experiencing significant sleep-related impairment. This underscores the importance of clinical judgement and patient-centered care in treatment planning.

In research, there is a growing call for sleep to be treated not just as a side issue, but as a core domain in PCNS assessment and intervention. Objective studies using actigraphy, polysomnography, and biomarker analysis are needed to understand the specific nature of sleep disruption in this population. Importantly, sleep quality should also be considered a key outcome measure in trials evaluating treatments for PCNS.

In summary, sleep disturbance is a central and disabling feature of PCNS. It reflects complex neurological, immunological, and psychological interactions that are still being unraveled. It worsens nearly every other symptom and undermines recovery, yet it remains under-assessed, under-treated, and often misunderstood. Addressing sleep in PCNS is not optional it is essential. Restoring restorative sleep is a critical step toward restoring lives.

3.5.7 Autonomic Nervous System Dysfunction and PCNS: When the Body's Regulation Breaks Down

Dysautonomia, or dysfunction of the autonomic nervous system (ANS), is increasingly recognized as a prominent feature of Post-COVID-19 Neurological Syndrome (PCNS). The ANS regulates many of the body's involuntary functions heart rate, blood pressure, temperature control, digestion, and respiratory rhythm. When this system becomes dysregulated, the effects are felt throughout the body.

In patients with PCNS, signs of dysautonomia may appear early, during the acute phase of COVID-19 infection, or they may develop weeks to months later. Symptoms vary in severity and presentation, but they often include orthostatic intolerance (difficulty standing), palpitations, dizziness, gastrointestinal disturbances, temperature sensitivity, and profound fatigue. These symptoms are not only distressing they are disabling. For many, they fluctuate day to day or even hour to hour, making daily functioning unpredictable.

One patient described her experience:

> Some days I can walk fine. Other days, I faint standing up. My heart races after I eat. I don't trust my own body anymore.

This sense of bodily betrayal is common. For people who previously led active, independent lives, the sudden loss of internal stability can be frightening and life-altering.

3.5.8 Understanding the Autonomic Nervous System in PCNS

The autonomic nervous system is divided into two branches: the sympathetic nervous system (which activates the fight-or-flight response) and the parasympathetic nervous system (which promotes rest and recovery). In healthy individuals, these systems work together to maintain physiological balance. In PCNS, however, this coordination appears disrupted.

Emerging evidence suggests that SARS-CoV-2 can trigger a cascade of immune-mediated changes that affect the autonomic nervous system. These include direct viral invasion of nerve tissue, autoimmune responses against autonomic ganglia, and widespread neuroinflammation. In addition, damage to the small nerve fibers responsible for regulating autonomic functions known as small fiber neuropathy has been reported in people with PCNS, further supporting the biological basis of dysautonomia in this population.

3.6 Postural Orthostatic Tachycardia Syndrome (POTS)

Among the various forms of dysautonomia, Postural Orthostatic Tachycardia Syndrome (POTS) has emerged as a common and particularly disabling condition in PCNS patients. POTS is characterized by an excessive increase in heart rate (more than 30 beats/min in adults, or more than 40 in adolescents) within 10 min of standing, without a corresponding drop in blood pressure.

The typical symptoms include lightheadedness, palpitations, shortness of breath, chest discomfort, shakiness, nausea, and even episodes of near-fainting or actual syncope. These symptoms are typically relieved by lying down, but can return quickly upon standing or walking.

Many PCNS patients meet criteria for POTS but remain undiagnosed due to limited awareness of the condition among clinicians. This often leads to misdiagnosis as anxiety, panic disorder, or deconditioning. In reality, POTS is a measurable physiological disorder that requires targeted management.

In clinical settings, a simple active stand test or a formal tilt-table test can confirm the diagnosis. Once identified, POTS can be treated through a combination of lifestyle adjustments, fluid and salt intake, compression garments, and medications such as beta-blockers, fludrocortisone, or ivabradine. However, treatment must be individualized and delivered with a clear understanding of the underlying dysautonomia.

3.7 Impact on Daily Life and Function

Dysautonomia in PCNS is not only medically significant it is deeply disruptive. The symptoms are unpredictable, often coming in waves, and may not be visible to others. Patients may look well while seated, but experience intense symptoms when standing, moving, or even digesting a meal. This invisibility contributes to stigma and misunderstanding.

For many, dysautonomia interferes with essential activities: walking, working, cooking, shopping, and socializing. Some are unable to stand long enough to take a shower. Others must rest for hours after light exertion. One young adult who was previously a long-distance runner now uses a wheelchair to leave the house, due to severe orthostatic intolerance.

This loss of function leads to secondary challenges. Social isolation, loss of employment, reduced income, and dependence on caregivers are common. The psychological toll is considerable. Feelings of helplessness, frustration, and grief for a previous life are widespread, especially when symptoms are dismissed or misunderstood by healthcare providers.

3.8 Diagnostic Challenges and Clinical Misunderstanding

Unfortunately, dysautonomia remains underdiagnosed in the PCNS population. Standard blood tests and imaging studies are often normal. When patients describe their symptoms especially those involving heart palpitations, chest discomfort, or faintness they are frequently referred to cardiologists or psychiatrists. Many undergo extensive testing without conclusive results, or worse, are told that their symptoms are "just anxiety."

This misunderstanding stems from a lack of training in autonomic disorders. Few medical curricula include dedicated teaching on dysautonomia, and even fewer include hands-on training in how to assess it. As a result, patients are left in diagnostic limbo, sometimes for years.

To address this gap, clinicians must be educated to recognize dysautonomia as a neurological condition with a clear set of signs, symptoms, and diagnostic criteria. A structured autonomic screening protocol should be incorporated into the routine assessment of patients with PCNS. Questions about standing tolerance, meal-induced symptoms, temperature sensitivity, and GI dysmotility should be standard.

3.9 Management Strategies

Managing dysautonomia in PCNS requires a comprehensive and individualized approach. Non-pharmacological strategies are the first line and include:

- Increasing fluid intake to 2–3 l/day
- Liberal use of dietary salt (unless contraindicated)
- Wearing abdominal binders or compression stockings
- Elevating the head of the bed to prevent overnight blood pooling
- Engaging in recumbent or semi-recumbent exercise (e.g., recumbent biking, swimming)

When these are insufficient, medications can help stabilize autonomic tone and reduce symptoms. These may include:

- Beta-blockers to reduce heart rate
- Fludrocortisone to expand blood volume
- Midodrine to raise blood pressure
- Ivabradine to slow heart rate without lowering blood pressure

Access to multidisciplinary teams including neurologists, cardiologists, physiotherapists, and occupational therapists is ideal. However, such care is not available in many settings, particularly in rural or low-resource areas. In these cases, telehealth and patient-led education resources can play a critical role.

3.10 The Path Forward

Dysautonomia in PCNS is real, measurable, and debilitating. It deserves greater clinical recognition, better diagnostic tools, and dedicated research. We must move beyond vague labels and outdated assumptions and begin to see this for what it is: a complex neurological condition that undermines basic functions of life.

Importantly, dysautonomia is not a stand-alone issue. It intersects with fatigue, brain fog, sleep disturbance, and emotional regulation—all key features of PCNS. By identifying and addressing dysautonomia, clinicians can help reduce the overall burden of the syndrome and support better quality of life.

Recognizing POTS and other forms of autonomic dysfunction as part of the PCNS spectrum is not just medically accurate it is an act of validation. For patients who have spent months or years searching for answers, that recognition is the first step toward recovery.

3.11 Anxiety, Depression, and Emotional Dysregulation: A Secondary Burden, or a Core Symptom?

The emotional consequences of Post-COVID-19 Neurological Syndrome (PCNS) are profound. For many, the experience of living with PCNS is not just defined by cognitive issues, fatigue, or autonomic dysfunction, but also by overwhelming emotional distress. While some mental health symptoms appear to arise in response to prolonged illness and disability, growing evidence suggests that mood disturbances—such as anxiety, depression, and emotional instability—are primary components of the syndrome itself.

Patients frequently describe changes in their emotional responses that feel foreign and involuntary. Emotional outbursts, panic attacks, tearfulness without warning, and feelings of detachment or emptiness are commonly reported. One woman who had never previously experienced mood disorders put it simply:

> I used to be a strong, happy person. Now I cry for no reason and feel like I'm watching life happen from behind glass.

These symptoms are not merely psychological reactions to illness. Increasingly, research points to biological underpinnings. Neuroinflammation, disruptions in neurotransmitter signaling, and direct or immune-mediated effects on brain structures like the limbic system and prefrontal cortex are thought to contribute to mood dysregulation in PCNS. Functional MRI studies and CSF analyses from post-COVID cohorts have identified alterations in brain metabolism and inflammatory markers associated with emotional control, suggesting that the emotional manifestations of PCNS are as neurological as they are psychological.

3.11.1 Anxiety: More Than a Reaction

Anxiety is one of the most frequently reported emotional symptoms in PCNS. This can take the form of generalized anxiety, social anxiety, or panic attacks. Many patients describe sudden episodes of racing thoughts, heart palpitations, chest tightness, and a sense of impending doom. For some, these symptoms appear during or after exertion. For others, they strike at random, including during sleep.

What distinguishes PCNS-related anxiety from primary anxiety disorders is the context. Many patients have no prior history of anxiety. The symptom onset is sudden and coincides with other neurological symptoms. It may also be exacerbated by dysautonomia, which causes similar physiological sensations (e.g., tachycardia, shortness of breath), making the anxiety feel somatic and inescapable.

A key concern is that this anxiety is often misattributed as the cause of PCNS symptoms rather than a symptom itself. This misattribution leads to delays in appropriate care, reinforces patient stigma, and undermines trust in the healthcare system.

3.11.2 Depression and Affective Flattening

Depressive symptoms in PCNS can range from low mood and apathy to full episodes of major depressive disorder. Patients report a loss of interest in previously enjoyed activities, social withdrawal, sleep disturbances, feelings of worthlessness, and thoughts of hopelessness. In many cases, these symptoms emerge in parallel with physical decline and loss of functional ability, particularly among individuals who are no longer able to work, parent, or participate in normal routines.

Beyond classic depression, some individuals experience affective flattening or emotional blunting a reduced capacity to feel emotional highs and lows. This state of numbness can be deeply unsettling. One patient described it as "being alive but not connected," unable to cry, laugh, or feel joy even in moments that would have previously brought strong emotion.

Neurobiologically, depression in PCNS may be linked to changes in serotonin and dopamine pathways, altered hypothalamic-pituitary-adrenal (HPA) axis function, and inflammation-driven damage to circuits involved in reward and motivation.

3.11.3 Emotional Dysregulation: A Neurological Symptom

Emotional dysregulation rapid mood swings, increased irritability, and heightened sensitivity is another common feature in PCNS. Patients often report feeling as though they are on an emotional rollercoaster. Minor stressors can trigger exaggerated emotional reactions. Some describe sudden crying spells, anger outbursts, or an inability to "calm down" once emotionally activated.

This lability is characteristic of neurological disorders involving frontal-limbic circuit dysfunction. In PCNS, these symptoms may reflect damage or dysregulation in brain areas responsible for emotional control and executive function. They also appear to be worsened by sleep deprivation, hormonal fluctuations, and autonomic instability all common in PCNS.

3.11.4 Impact on Identity and Relationships

Living with emotional symptoms that feel unpredictable and foreign can erode a person's sense of self. Patients report feeling like strangers to their own emotions. Relationships suffer as mood instability leads to misunderstandings, withdrawal, or conflict. Partners, children, and close friends may struggle to understand the changes, particularly when outward physical signs of illness are minimal.

The inability to express or control emotion also creates internal conflict. Many patients experience guilt over how they respond to others or frustration with themselves for not being able to "get back to normal." These emotional burdens, when combined with physical symptoms, create a total-body syndrome that affects mind, function, and identity.

3.11.5 Barriers to Recognition and Care

One of the most damaging misconceptions about PCNS-related mood symptoms is that they are "just psychological." This language implies that the emotional disturbances are imaginary, exaggerated, or self-inflicted. It ignores the robust evidence of neurobiological changes and the systemic effects of chronic illness.

As a result, many patients are denied appropriate care. They are referred only for psychiatric evaluation, offered simplistic advice like "try to relax," or given medications without holistic support. Others are told to wait it out. Meanwhile, their quality of life continues to deteriorate.

There is an urgent need to reframe emotional symptoms in PCNS as integral, biologically mediated aspects of the syndrome. Doing so will help shift clinical attitudes, reduce stigma, and promote interdisciplinary care that includes neurologists, psychiatrists, psychologists, and rehabilitation professionals.

3.11.6 Treatment Considerations

Treating emotional symptoms in PCNS requires a personalized and compassionate approach. Some patients benefit from standard treatments for depression and anxiety, including selective serotonin reuptake inhibitors (SSRIs), serotonin-norepinephrine reuptake inhibitors (SNRIs), and cognitive behavioral therapy (CBT). However, others experience side effects or limited benefit, particularly when their emotional symptoms are tightly linked to other PCNS features like fatigue or dysautonomia.

Mind-body practices such as mindfulness, gentle movement, breathwork, and trauma-informed therapy can support regulation of both emotional and autonomic systems. Psychoeducation is also essential helping patients and their families understand that emotional changes are not a character flaw, but a symptom of a complex neurological condition.

Peer support, online communities, and guided recovery programs offer additional sources of validation and coping strategies. Access to these resources is critical, especially for those who feel isolated or dismissed in traditional healthcare settings.

3.11.7 Conclusion: Emotion as a Signal, Not a Distraction

The emotional burden of PCNS is not an afterthought. It is not secondary. It is not a side effect of "overreacting." It is a central component of the syndrome one that arises from both biological injury and the lived trauma of losing health, function, and certainty.

Recognizing anxiety, depression, and emotional dysregulation as core symptoms of PCNS allows us to respond more effectively, both clinically and socially. It opens the door to integrated care, patient validation, and long-term recovery strategies, and it reminds us that every emotional symptom is not a distraction from the real illness but a powerful signal of its depth and complexity.

3.12 Putting It All Together: A Syndrome That Disrupts Identity

PCNS is not one problem. It's many. It doesn't follow a single pattern, and it doesn't fit neatly into existing boxes, but its neurological core is clear. The brain is at the center of these dysfunctions cognitive, emotional, autonomic, and sensory.

What's perhaps most tragic is the way PCNS erodes a person's identity. People who once thrived parents, professionals, students, athletes suddenly find themselves housebound, dependent, and afraid. They feel dismissed by doctors and invisible to society.

We cannot continue to ignore this condition or minimize it with vague labels. The constellation of symptoms described here deserves a unified name, a dedicated care pathway, and a place in our public health systems. PCNS is real, measurable, and treatable if we choose to act.

3.13 Epidemiology and the GBD Framework

A large global analysis of over 1.2 million people from 22 countries has confirmed that a significant number of individuals continue to experience symptoms long after their initial COVID-19 illness. Using data from 54 studies and two large medical record databases, researchers found that about 6.2% of people with symptomatic SARS-CoV-2 infection developed at least one of three key symptom clusters: persistent fatigue with pain or mood changes, ongoing breathing issues, or cognitive problems such as brain fog. These symptoms were more common in women over 20 years of age, with nearly 11% affected, compared to about 5% of men. Younger people under 20 also experienced symptoms, but less often—around 2.8%. The duration of symptoms varied, with hospitalized patients experiencing an average of 9 months of symptoms and nonhospitalized individuals about 4 months. Alarmingly, 15% of those with Long COVID symptoms still had them a full year later, reinforcing that this is a chronic condition for many and not just a temporary phase [8]. The Global Burden of Disease (GBD) framework, coordinated by the Institute for Health Metrics and Evaluation (IHME), offers a global lens on disease impact through metrics such as Years Lived with Disability (YLD) and Disability-Adjusted Life Years (DALYs). However, PCNS is not yet recognized as a discrete condition within GBD classifications.

Using proxy indicators and modelled estimates:

- An estimated *150 million* people globally may experience PCNS.
- The *working-age population* (*30–59 years*) bears the highest burden.

- YLDs attributable to PCNS symptoms particularly fatigue, cognitive impairment, and mood disorders may exceed *20 million globally*.

Failure to identify PCNS within GBD models leads to underestimation of neurological burden and inadequate allocation of resources.

3.14 Overview of the Global Burden

A comprehensive Bayesian meta-regression analysis incorporating ten longitudinal cohort studies, two large U.S. medical record databases, and 44 peer-reviewed publications found that:

- An estimated *144.7 million people* globally experienced long COVID in 2020 and 2021.
- This accounts for roughly *3.7%* of all SARS-CoV-2 infections.
- The three main symptom clusters were:
  - *Fatigue*: present in ~51% of long COVID cases
  - *Cognitive dysfunction* (e.g., brain fog): in ~35%
  - *Respiratory symptoms*: in ~60%

Patients who were hospitalized during their acute infection tended to have more severe and longer-lasting symptoms. Median recovery times were nearly 9 months for hospitalized cases versus 4 months for community-based cases. Notably, about 15% of patients still reported symptoms at 12 months, signaling a chronic condition for many.

3.15 LMIC-Specific Considerations

While high-income countries (HICs) may be better equipped to measure, diagnose, and treat long COVID, LMICs face data gaps and limited capacity for ongoing care. Surveillance systems in many LMICs were overwhelmed during the height of the pandemic and are often not equipped to track long-term outcomes. Additionally, in LMICs, the overlap between long COVID symptoms and endemic diseases (e.g., tuberculosis, malnutrition, chronic fatigue from vector-borne infections) complicates diagnosis.

Health systems in LMICs often lack trained rehabilitation specialists, neurologists, and respiratory therapists. As a result, patients are frequently referred between specialties or denied treatment entirely. This “invisible” burden disproportionately affects working-age adults and women, deepening existing inequalities.

A key finding from the GBD-aligned modeling was the use of severity-weighted prevalence (similar to Years Lived with Disability or YLDs). In LMICs, the severity-weighted burden of long COVID may be even more significant due to compounding factors such as poor baseline health, delayed care, and lower health literacy.

3.16 Regional Burden and Inequity

Using extrapolated GBD data, we find that PCNS disproportionately affects populations in:

- *South Asia* (40+ million cases)
- *Sub-Saharan Africa* (20+ million cases)
- *Latin America* (19 million cases)

Low- and middle-income countries (LMICs) face compounded challenges: poor diagnostic infrastructure, limited neurology workforce, and competing health priorities.

3.17 Disability and Economic Consequences (Table 3.2)

PCNS is a leading cause of long-term disability among COVID-19 survivors:

- Cognitive and autonomic symptoms limit return to work.
- Affected individuals report lost income, employment instability, and reduced quality of life.
- Women are disproportionately affected, reflecting gendered disparities in both exposure and caregiving responsibilities.

Table 3.2 Gaps in surveillance and policy response for PCNS

Domain	Current status	Recommendation
ICD Classification	PCNS not recognized as a standalone entity	Advocate for inclusion in ICD-11
GBD Inclusion	No separate code or burden estimation	Model PCNS as a unique post-viral syndrome
National Health Strategies	Rarely acknowledged in COVID recovery plans	Integrate into long COVID and NCD strategies
Data Infrastructure	Limited long-term neurological tracking	Invest in longitudinal registries
LMIC Support	Minimal access to neurological services	Build local neurorehab and brain health capacity

3.18 Why the Name Matters: PCNS Over Long COVID

The term "*Long COVID*" is diffuse and often misunderstood. It fails to convey the specificity and severity of the brain-related impacts. Adopting *Post-COVID-19 Neurological Syndrome* (*PCNS*):

- Emphasizes the neurological underpinnings
- Supports dedicated research and care pathways
- Improves diagnostic clarity and patient validation

Recognizing PCNS in ICD and GBD classifications will drive much-needed funding, workforce development, and policy integration.

3.19 Recommendations

1. *Formal recognition of PCNS* in WHO ICD-11 and GBD disease taxonomies
2. *Development of consensus clinical criteria* through neurology societies and rehabilitation networks
3. *Establishment of PCNS clinics* in both high-income and low-resource settings
4. *Dedicated funding streams* for PCNS research, including biomarker development and rehabilitation outcomes
5. *Global surveillance mechanisms* to track PCNS cases and outcomes over time

3.20 Conclusion

Post-COVID-19 Neurological Syndrome (PCNS) is real, disabling, and measurable. It affects millions and will continue to shape the global neurological burden for decades. By recognizing PCNS as a standalone neurological condition, we can align clinical, research, and policy efforts to address this silent epidemic and support those who live with it.

Further Reading

1. Wijeratne T, Crewther S. Post-COVID-19 neurological syndrome (PCNS); a novel syndrome with challenges for the global neurology community. J Neurol Sci. 2020;419:117179.
2. Vos T, et al. Global burden of 369 diseases and injuries in 204 countries and territories. Lancet. 2020;396:1204–22.
3. Institute for Health Metrics and Evaluation (IHME). Global burden of disease 2021: findings from the GBD 2021 study. Seattle. WA: IHME, 2024.
4. Australian Parliament House. Sick and tired: casting a long shadow—inquiry into long COVID and repeated COVID infections. 2023. https://www.aph.gov.au/.../Chapter_4_-_Lived_experiences_of_long_COVID.

5. Soriano JB, et al. A clinical case definition of post-COVID-19 condition by a Delphi consensus. Lancet Infect Dis. 2022;22:e102–7.
6. Institute for Health Metrics and Evaluation (IHME). About GBD. Seattle: IHME; 2024. Available at: https://www.healthdata.org/research-analysis/about-gbd. Accessed 20 May 2025.
7. World Health Organization (WHO). Global health estimates: leading causes of DALYs. Geneva: WHO; 2023. Available at: https://www.who.int/data/gho/data/themes/mortality-and-global-health-estimates/global-health-estimates-leading-causes-of-dalys. Accessed 20 May 2025.
8. Hanson SW, Abbafati C, Aerts JG, Al-Aly Z, Ashbaugh C, Ballouz T, et al. Estimated global proportions of individuals with persistent fatigue, cognitive, and respiratory symptoms following symptomatic COVID-19: a Bayesian meta-regression analysis. JAMA. 2022;328(16):1604–15. Available at: https://jamanetwork.com/journals/jama/fullarticle/2797443. Accessed 20 May 2025.
9. Murray CJL, Lopez AD, IHME COVID-19 Forecasting Team. The burden of long COVID: global estimates and implications. Scholars@Duke. 2023. Available at: https://scholars.duke.edu/individual/pub1524278. Accessed 20 May 2025.
10. The Lancet COVID-19 Commission. The global impact of COVID-19 and strategies for LMICs. The Lancet. 2021;398(10295):1525–76. Available at: https://www.thelancet.com/journals/lancet/article/PIIS0140-6736%2821%2902444-2/fulltext. Accessed 20 May 2025.

4 Post-COVID-19 Neurological Syndrome and the WHO Intersectoral Global Action Plan

Reuben Parama Iswara and Tissa Wijeratne

Neurological disorders now account for more disability-adjusted life years (DALYs) than any other disease category worldwide. The World Health Organization (WHO), through its *Intersectoral Global Action Plan on Epilepsy and Other Neurological Disorders* (*IGAP*) 2022–2031, has acknowledged the urgent need to address this escalating burden with coordinated, cross-sectoral strategies. IGAP's central vision is a world where brain health is valued, promoted, and protected across the life course and where individuals living with neurological disorders can access timely diagnosis, treatment, care, and support, free from stigma and discrimination [1].

One of the emerging yet insufficiently recognized contributors to the global neurological burden is *Post-COVID-19 Neurological Syndrome* (PCNS) [2, 3]. This chapter introduces PCNS not as an incidental outcome of the COVID-19 pandemic, but as a standalone neurological disorder that demands integration into the IGAP framework. It presents a strong case for inclusion of PCNS in national neurological strategies, underpinned by clinical, epidemiological, and patient-reported evidence, and aligned with IGAP's goals of improving care access, reducing disability, and safeguarding the rights of affected individuals.

While the acute threat of COVID-19 has receded in many parts of the world, its neurological legacy continues to unfold. PCNS affects millions globally, with symptoms that impair cognition, emotion, mobility, and autonomic regulation, yet it remains absent from most formal disease classifications, health system plans, and burden of disease estimates. As a result, people living with PCNS often face

R. Parama Iswara (✉)
Department of Neurology, Western Health, Melbourne, VIC, Australia
e-mail: Reuben.ParamaIswara@wh.org.au

T. Wijeratne
Department of Neurology and Stroke, La Trobe University, St. Albans, VIC, Australia
e-mail: tissa.wijeratne@wh.org.au

T. Wijeratne, S. Crewther (eds.), *Post Covid-19 Neurological Syndrome*,
https://doi.org/10.1007/978-3-032-14995-4_4

fragmented care pathways, delayed diagnoses, and significant psychosocial and economic hardship.

The WHO IGAP was developed precisely to address these systemic gaps. With ten global targets and five core strategic objectives, the plan sets a roadmap for countries to integrate neurological conditions into their health and social service frameworks. The recently released *WHO IGAP Implementation Toolkit* provides practical actions for national and regional actors, including ministries of health, civil society organizations, clinicians, and people with lived experience. It emphasizes stakeholder engagement, situational analysis, and the development of integrated service delivery models.

In this chapter, we use the structure and tools offered by IGAP and its Toolkit as a framework to explore how the needs of PCNS patients can be addressed at scale. We highlight five priority areas where alignment with IGAP is both possible and essential:

1. *Policy and Governance Integration*

   We demonstrate why PCNS should be incorporated into national neurological health plans. Its multisystemic nature aligns with IGAP's call for a life-course, person-centered approach that integrates neurology into broader health and social policies.
2. *Diagnosis, Treatment, and Care Pathways*

   We review evidence showing the significant care gap for PCNS patients and recommend strategies based on IGAP's guidance for scaling up neurological workforce capacity, improving diagnostic access, and delivering multidisciplinary care.
3. *Promotion of Brain Health and Prevention*

   We argue that public awareness of PCNS must increase if stigma is to be reduced and early identification improved. Preventive strategies must address high-risk populations and mitigate long-term disability, particularly in underserved regions.
4. *Strengthening Research and Information Systems*

   We advocate for the inclusion of PCNS in surveillance systems and burden of disease metrics (such as the Global Burden of Disease study). This is vital to track the true impact of PCNS and drive equitable funding for research and care innovation.
5. *Advocacy, Inclusion, and Human Rights*

   PCNS has disproportionately affected working-age individuals, many of whom are now unemployed or socially marginalized. We examine the human rights dimensions of PCNS and the importance of involving people with lived experience in policy-making and service design.

The WHO IGAP Toolkit urges countries to adopt an integrated approach to neurological care, emphasizing that brain health must be protected from childhood through old age, and that neurological services should be embedded within primary health care, mental health services, and public health systems. This is particularly relevant for PCNS, whose symptoms cut across neurology, psychiatry, rehabilitation, and internal medicine. Traditional, siloed models of care cannot meet the complex needs of these patients.

Moreover, the toolkit's insistence on stakeholder engagement and co-design with people living with neurological disorders is especially pertinent. PCNS patients have been instrumental in shaping public discourse, yet they continue to report invalidation and neglect in clinical settings. Their stories, many of which are drawn from national inquiries such as the Australian Federal Parliament's 2023 Long COVID report, reveal the human cost of a fragmented response. Recognizing PCNS through an IGAP lens offers a way to center their voices in policy and service development.

The lack of formal disease coding for PCNS further limits progress. Without recognition in systems like the ICD-11 or explicit inclusion in UHC benefit packages, patients are left to navigate complex symptoms without access to specialist care, rehabilitation services, or social support. This represents not only a treatment gap, but also an "inclusion gap"—a concept highlighted in IGAP to describe the systemic exclusion of people with neurological disorders from mainstream health and social systems.

Finally, this chapter connects PCNS with broader global goals. Addressing PCNS through the IGAP framework contributes directly to the Sustainable Development Goals (SDGs)—particularly those related to health (SDG 3), poverty reduction (SDG 1), education (SDG 4), and gender equality (SDG 5). By reducing the neurological burden of COVID-19, we can mitigate long-term economic impacts, support workforce re-entry, and prevent health systems from becoming overwhelmed by chronic post-viral sequelae.

In summary, this chapter serves as both a call to action and a guide. We advocate for the formal recognition of PCNS as a neurological disorder, fully aligned with the WHO IGAP. We outline how countries can use the IGAP Toolkit to integrate PCNS into policy, service delivery, and research agendas. Through case studies, patient vignettes, epidemiological modeling, and implementation strategies, we aim to provide a comprehensive roadmap for responding to this growing public health challenge.

PCNS is not just a post-pandemic inconvenience, it is a long-term neurological condition that now affects tens of millions. Without deliberate, evidence-informed action, it risks becoming one of the defining neglected disorders of our time. IGAP gives us the tools to act. The time to use them is now.

4.1 Policy and Governance Integration: Making PCNS Visible in National Neurological Strategies

The global pandemic has left behind a lasting neurological shadow. Post-COVID-19 Neurological Syndrome (PCNS) represents a growing, unmet need across health systems worldwide, yet it remains largely invisible in current policies. Despite its substantial burden impacting cognition, mood, autonomic stability, and functional independence. PCNS has not been formally incorporated into most national neurological strategies. This omission reflects a deeper issue: the historical marginalization of neurological disorders in health policy, now echoed in the post-COVID landscape.

The WHO Intersectoral Global Action Plan (IGAP) provides an opportunity to change that trajectory. Its call for the full integration of neurological conditions into health policy across the life course creates the ideal policy window to incorporate PCNS into national planning. Under IGAP's first strategic objective to strengthen governance and leadership. Countries are encouraged to develop or revise national neurological health plans to be inclusive, person-centered, and data-driven. PCNS must be included in these frameworks if the needs of millions of affected individuals are to be addressed.

4.1.1 A Multisystemic Disorder, Requiring Multisectoral Governance

PCNS, by its very nature, is multisystemic. It blurs the traditional lines between neurology, psychiatry, internal medicine, immunology, and rehabilitation. This complexity makes it difficult to manage using disease-specific approaches. Instead, a comprehensive, whole-of-system response is needed one that aligns with IGAP's vision of integrating neurological care into broader health and social systems, education, workforce development, and universal health coverage.

For example, individuals living with PCNS often face challenges accessing appropriate care because their symptoms fall across multiple specialties. Cognitive dysfunction may lead to a neurology referral, emotional dysregulation may result in psychiatric evaluation, fatigue may be dismissed as psychological, and autonomic symptoms may be misattributed to anxiety. As a result, patients are frequently caught in a web of fragmented, uncoordinated care. This not only delays diagnosis but also increases the risk of chronic disability.

A national neurological plan that explicitly includes PCNS can begin to address these silos. Such a plan should outline clinical pathways that account for the multisystem presentation of PCNS, promote interdisciplinary care models, and facilitate timely access to rehabilitation and support services. It should also enable case finding, early intervention, and continuity of care across health settings.

4.1.2 Aligning with the Life-Course Approach

One of the core principles of IGAP is the life-course approach recognizing that brain health must be protected and promoted from prenatal development through to old age. PCNS disproportionately affects working-age adults, many of whom were previously healthy and economically active. These individuals often fall through the gaps of existing neurological care models, which may focus more heavily on age-related neurodegenerative conditions.

By integrating PCNS into national neurological strategies, countries can apply a life-course lens that captures these mid-life neurological disruptions. This would allow for improved tracking, workforce support, and long-term planning ensuring that services evolve to meet the changing profile of neurological disability in the post-pandemic era.

Furthermore, including PCNS in national strategies provides a path to equity. Studies consistently show that people from lower socio-economic backgrounds, women, and ethnic minorities are disproportionately affected by Long COVID, including PCNS. A governance structure that identifies these disparities and embeds targeted interventions is critical. This aligns with IGAP's emphasis on equity and inclusion in neurological policy-making.

4.1.3 From National Plans to Funded Action

Incorporating PCNS into policy is not just about language. It must lead to action. National neurological plans that recognize PCNS must be backed by resourced implementation plans. This includes:

- Funding for research and data collection on PCNS prevalence, outcomes, and care gaps.
- Inclusion of PCNS in national surveillance and electronic health record coding systems.
- Investment in workforce development, including training for primary care providers and specialists.
- Establishment of referral networks that support integrated, multidisciplinary care.
- Development of public health campaigns to increase awareness and reduce stigma.

Each of these actions is aligned with the WHO IGAP Toolkit, which outlines practical, context-sensitive measures for implementing national plans. The Toolkit emphasizes the importance of tailoring strategies to country-specific priorities and leveraging existing infrastructure. For PCNS, this may mean integrating care pathways into Long COVID clinics, leveraging stroke or rehabilitation programs, and co-locating services within primary care or mental health settings.

4.1.4 Leveraging Existing Structures and Partnerships

The COVID-19 pandemic led many countries to establish taskforces, clinics, and registries for Long COVID. While these efforts are commendable, they have often developed in parallel to national neurological services. To build a sustainable response, PCNS must now be bridged into existing neurological governance structures.

This integration requires collaboration between ministries of health, neurology societies, patient organizations, and public health agencies. National neurological councils or steering groups should include representatives from PCNS-affected communities, as well as clinicians who have treated these patients. These stakeholders can guide the incorporation of PCNS into national guidelines, workforce strategies, and monitoring frameworks.

International partnerships also play a role. Multilateral support from WHO, regional neurological federations, and global health donors can assist countries in developing PCNS-inclusive neurological strategies, especially in low- and middle-income settings where resources are constrained. Advocacy networks and patient-led initiatives must also be resourced to ensure that those most affected are included in decision-making.

4.1.5 Recognizing PCNS in Global Classification Systems

A critical governance issue is the current lack of formal disease classification for PCNS in systems such as the International Classification of Diseases (ICD-11). Without diagnostic codes, PCNS remains invisible in national health data, insurance systems, and research registries. This invisibility undermines policy planning, resource allocation, and the development of care pathways.

National neurological plans must therefore advocate for PCNS to be formally recognized in global classification systems. This will enable standardized coding, better tracking, and inclusion in disability and mortality statistics. It will also facilitate access to social protection and disability benefits for affected individuals.

4.1.6 Conclusion: Policy Inclusion Is the First Step toward Health Justice

Integrating PCNS into national neurological plans is not merely a technical exercise—it is a matter of health justice. By formally recognizing PCNS as a neurological condition within policy frameworks, countries can acknowledge the suffering of millions, mobilize coordinated responses, and bring legitimacy to a neglected disorder.

The WHO IGAP and its Implementation Toolkit provide a ready-made framework for action. They offer tools, principles, and examples that countries can adapt to include PCNS in their health governance systems, but it requires political will, cross-sectoral collaboration, and patient engagement.

As countries revise or develop their national neurological action plans over the coming years, PCNS must be on the agenda. If we fail to integrate it now, we risk repeating the same exclusion that has long hindered progress in neurology. If we succeed, we lay the groundwork for a more responsive, equitable, and person-centered health system. One that truly reflects the full spectrum of neurological need in the twenty-first century.

4.2 Diagnosis, Treatment, and Care Pathways: From Recognition to Real Response

One of the most urgent and preventable failures in global health policy today is the continued reluctance to formally name and address *Post-COVID-19 Neurological Syndrome (PCNS)* as the distinct neurological condition it is. Instead, the umbrella term "Post COVID-19 condition" continues to dominate clinical documentation, public communication, and health system coding. While the intention may have been to offer flexibility, in practice this imprecision has led to fragmentation of care, confusion among providers, and prolonged suffering for patients.

The failure to recognize PCNS for what it is—a multisystem neurological disorder—has real consequences. People with debilitating symptoms are turned away from specialist care, told their symptoms are too vague, or inappropriately routed to psychiatric services. Clinicians, uncertain about guidelines or diagnostic frameworks, may defer to exclusionary tests rather than holistic evaluation. Meanwhile, national health systems miss the opportunity to scale up targeted care, conduct research, or plan for long-term rehabilitation.

It is time to stop going around in circles with vague labels. The people experiencing disabling neurological symptoms after COVID-19 do not have a generic "post-viral malaise." They have a syndrome that fits squarely within neurology—a syndrome that affects memory, cognition, autonomic function, emotion, pain perception, and physical stamina. Naming it PCNS is not only clinically accurate—it is necessary for diagnosis, treatment, and systems planning.

4.2.1 The Care Gap

The current gap between need and care for PCNS patients is enormous. Data from high-income and low-resource settings alike show that individuals with PCNS symptoms often wait months to be seen, if they are seen at all. Many never receive a formal diagnosis. Only a minority access specialized neurology or rehabilitation services, and fewer still receive coordinated, multidisciplinary care.

A recent analysis of Long COVID clinics in the UK and USA found that neurological complaints—including brain fog, headaches, dizziness, and paresthesia—were among the most frequent but least understood symptoms reported. Despite this, only a small proportion of patients were referred to neurologists. The majority were instead routed through general medicine, psychiatry, or post-viral fatigue pathways, with little cross-specialty communication.

This lack of clear pathways reflects the broader problem: without specific recognition of PCNS, there are no tailored clinical guidelines, no standardized triage models, and no workforce strategy to meet the rising demand.

4.2.2 IGAP's Call to Action

The WHO Intersectoral Global Action Plan (IGAP) provides an important corrective. Its guidance calls for the development of integrated, multidisciplinary care models for neurological disorders—grounded in a person-centered, life-course approach. IGAP explicitly encourages governments to build diagnostic and treatment infrastructure that reflects the real burden of neurological disease, rather than limiting services to a narrow range of conditions.

For PCNS, this means building dedicated care pathways that include:

- *Early identification protocols* in primary care settings
- *Rapid access to neurological evaluation*, including cognitive and autonomic assessment
- *Multidisciplinary team care*, including neurology, neuropsychology, rehabilitation, mental health, and primary care
- *Patient navigation and support services* to help individuals access ongoing care, employment services, and social protection

This is not theoretical. Countries already developing national neurological plans under IGAP are encouraged to use the WHO IGAP Implementation Toolkit, which offers a checklist and decision aids for integrating conditions like PCNS into service planning. One of the Toolkit's guiding principles is that conditions of emerging burden and unmet need must not be overlooked. PCNS fits this description precisely.

4.2.3 Diagnostic Challenges and Solutions

Diagnosing PCNS is not straightforward—but it is possible. It requires a syndromic approach informed by history, symptom clusters, functional impact, and exclusion of other acute causes, yet many health systems lack diagnostic algorithms or protocols for PCNS, and some still dismiss symptoms as anxiety or deconditioning.

Standard diagnostic workups often return normal findings, frustrating both patients and providers. This highlights the need for:

- *Functional and performance-based assessments* (e.g., cognitive batteries, orthostatic vitals)
- *Validated symptom checklists* to capture fluctuating, multi-domain issues
- *Standardized documentation* using consistent terminology, including formal codes when available
- *Training for clinicians*, especially general practitioners, on how to recognize and manage PCNS in the absence of conventional test abnormalities

Recognizing PCNS also allows for more precise health system coding. The current use of general "Post Acute COVID-19 condition" codes does little to track the real burden of neurological sequelae or monitor treatment outcomes. As ICD-11 evolves, explicit coding of PCNS should be advocated for, along with its inclusion in electronic health record templates, epidemiological surveys, and health insurance benefit packages.

4.2.4 Treatment and Management Models

Managing PCNS requires a nuanced, flexible approach tailored to the individual's symptom profile, severity, and context. There is no single cure, but there are proven interventions that reduce suffering and improve function. These include:

- *Rehabilitation therapies*, such as neurocognitive therapy, physiotherapy, and occupational therapy
- *Pharmacological support*, including medications for headache, sleep, autonomic symptoms, and mood disturbances
- *Pacing and energy management education*, especially for patients with post-exertional symptom exacerbation
- *Cognitive-behavioral interventions* to support coping, emotional regulation, and lifestyle adaptation
- *Social and occupational support*, including return-to-work planning and disability accommodations

Multidisciplinary clinics are an ideal model but may not be feasible in all settings. In resource-constrained environments, task-shifting and community-based rehabilitation may provide effective alternatives. Telehealth services, group-based therapy models, and nurse-led care coordination can also improve access and reduce costs.

4.2.5 Scaling the Neurology Workforce

One of the most critical challenges facing PCNS care delivery is the shortage of trained providers. Globally, there are fewer than one neurologist per 100,000 people in many low-income countries, and even in high-income regions, neurology waitlists are growing.

IGAP calls for urgent investment in workforce development, including:

- Training primary care providers to recognize and manage common neurological symptoms
- Expanding neurorehabilitation training for physiotherapists, psychologists, and nurses
- Developing clinical protocols and referral tools that reduce over-reliance on subspecialist access
- Leveraging e-learning, virtual consultations, and mobile health tools to scale expertise

For PCNS, workforce expansion must be rapid and creative. Integrating neurology into Long COVID care teams, retraining internal medicine providers, and supporting peer-to-peer clinical mentorship can increase capacity quickly while longer-term training programs evolve.

4.2.6 A Call for Honesty and Precision

There is no benefit in continuing to dilute the neurological reality of PCNS under vague terminology. Calling it "Post Acute COVID-19 condition" without naming its neurological nature confuses clinicians, misdirects patients, and weakens system-level responses. If this continues, the care gap will widen, data quality will suffer, and long-term disability will increase.

We must call PCNS what it is: a neurological syndrome with distinct features and measurable impact. By aligning diagnosis, treatment, and care planning with this clarity, health systems can begin to respond appropriately, and more importantly, compassionately.

4.3 Promotion of Brain Health and Prevention: The Critical Role of Public Awareness and Early Action for PCNS

Public health starts with recognition. For post-COVID-19 Neurological Syndrome (PCNS), the biggest challenge isn't a lack of suffering. It's a lack of visibility. People are living with disabling symptoms brain fog, fatigue, dizziness, autonomic instability, and mood changes but because the term "PCNS" is not commonly used in clinical settings, the condition is too often misunderstood, misclassified, or simply dismissed. To change this, we must increase public awareness and prioritize prevention and early intervention. This is not just about catching cases early. It's about protecting brain health across the lifespan and preserving quality of life for millions.

The WHO Intersectoral Global Action Plan (IGAP) calls for integrated strategies that promote brain health and prevent neurological disorders from early life to old age. PCNS fits squarely into this framework. Although triggered by a viral infection, its long-term effects are shaped by modifiable risk factors, inequities in access to care, and delays in recognition. Addressing PCNS through the lens of brain health promotion is not only feasible—it is essential.

4.3.1 Shifting the Narrative: From "Long COVID" to Brain Health

One of the major barriers to progress is the continued use of vague, generic terms like "Post COVID-19 condition." This phrase does not reflect the neurological core of what many patients experience. It leads to mislabelling of symptoms, fragmented care, and public confusion. Reframing this syndrome as a brain health issue, using the term *Post-COVID-19 Neurological Syndrome* indeed opens the door to education, advocacy, and early intervention.

Naming PCNS also shifts attention to prevention. If people understand that COVID-19 can result in long-lasting brain dysfunction, they are more likely to seek early care, prioritize recovery, and support public health measures to reduce transmission and improve post-viral monitoring. It also allows health systems to design messaging and screening tools that resonate with both patients and providers.

4.3.2 Promoting Brain Health: What We've Already Done

We are not starting from scratch. The global brain health community has already made strides in promoting prevention-focused initiatives that align with IGAP. One example is the *Life's Ten* framework, an evidence-based, lifestyle-driven approach to brain health that we have championed internationally. The Life's Ten principles include:

1. Eat healthy
2. Sleep healthy
3. Be physically active
4. Don't smoke
5. Manage stress better
6. Control blood sugar
7. Control blood pressure
8. Control lipids
9. Maintain a healthy abdominal circumference
10. Stay socially and mentally active

Each of these pillars has been shown to reduce the risk of neurological disorders, from stroke and dementia to migraine and now PCNS. While we cannot change the fact that someone has contracted COVID-19, we can reduce their risk of long-term complications by promoting better baseline brain health before, during, and after infection. Importantly, several of these principles directly mitigate the symptoms of PCNS, improving sleep, reducing anxiety, supporting cardiovascular and autonomic function, and restoring cognitive clarity.

We've also embedded these principles in community-based education and prevention campaigns. For example, our *World Brain Day 2023* campaign, co-led with the World Federation of Neurology, focused on "Brain Health and Disability Prevention." It reached millions globally with simple, clear messages about how to protect the brain throughout life, including in the post-infection period. Educational posters, webinars, school-based programs, and digital campaigns all helped spread the message that brain health matters, and that it's never too early, or too late, to act.

4.3.3 Why Prevention Matters for PCNS

The case for prevention in PCNS is strong. Research has shown that pre-existing conditions like diabetes, hypertension, obesity, and poor sleep are associated with more severe and longer-lasting post-COVID symptoms. Social isolation, psychological distress, and poor baseline mental health further increase vulnerability. These are all targets of prevention strategies.

By identifying and supporting high-risk populations—such as frontline workers, older adults, socioeconomically disadvantaged groups, and those with pre-existing neurological or mental health conditions—we can implement proactive strategies to monitor symptoms early, offer support quickly, and prevent disability.

This aligns closely with IGAP's call for "targeted prevention efforts for populations at higher risk of developing neurological disorders," especially in low- and middle-income countries (LMICs). In these settings, the pandemic has magnified existing health inequities. Without early education and brain health promotion, PCNS will continue to be overlooked, under-reported, and untreated.

4.3.4 The Role of Schools, Workplaces, and Primary Care

Promotion of brain health cannot be confined to hospitals or research centers. It must reach communities where people live, work, study, and socialize. In our recent initiatives, we've partnered with schools, municipal councils, and primary care providers to integrate brain health into everyday life.

In *Melton City Council*, Australia, we launched a brain health education program for high school students, focusing on lifestyle, sleep, digital habits, and early symptom recognition. These students learned not only how to protect their own brains, but how to identify signs of brain dysfunction in peers and family members, a crucial tool in the post-COVID world.

At the Australian Institute of Migraine, we've piloted education modules for primary care clinicians on identifying early signs of PCNS. These include brief screening tools, red flag symptoms, and guidance on when to refer. This front-line approach is key most PCNS patients first present in general practice, and many never make it to neurology unless primary care providers recognize the warning signs.

In the workplace, we've initiated wellness campaigns that blend mental health, physical health, and brain health under a unified umbrella. This holistic model makes prevention practical and accessible, especially for people who may otherwise normalize their symptoms or attribute them to stress or burnout.

The WHO IGAP Toolkit emphasizes the need to "raise awareness of the symptoms of neurological disorders in the general population and among healthcare professionals" as a foundational action. For PCNS, this is urgent. Too many patients remain undiagnosed for months, sometimes years, simply because they and their providers lack awareness.

Public campaigns must therefore focus on symptom recognition (e.g., persistent brain fog, post-exertional crashes, emotional instability, dizziness), care-seeking behavior, and destigmatization. At the same time, they should empower individuals to adopt brain-healthy behaviors, even before symptoms start [4–6]. This dual approach prevention plus early detection—is the key to reducing long-term disability.

We are also working to integrate PCNS messaging into existing stroke, dementia, and mental health platforms helping patients, families, and systems understand that PCNS is part of the broader brain health agenda. It is not an isolated anomaly. It is a continuation of what we already know: when the brain is inflamed, injured, or dysregulated, it needs care.

Promotion of brain health is not just a public health ideal. It is a practical strategy for reducing the burden of PCNS globally. By educating communities, supporting healthier lifestyles, identifying symptoms early, and reaching vulnerable populations, we can shift from a reactive to a proactive model.

The tools exist. The WHO IGAP Toolkit provides a clear pathway. Our work with Life's Ten, World Brain Day, and community-based programs shows that it can be done. What we need now is to embed these strategies into every national neurological plan, every recovery strategy, and every health communication campaign.

Preventing PCNS starts with believing it exists, educating the public, and recognizing that brain health is central to every individual's ability to live a full, connected life after COVID-19.

Post-COVID-19 Neurological Syndrome (PCNS) is real. It is disabling, and it is widespread, yet most countries still don't track it properly. It remains largely invisible in data systems, disease coding, and public health surveillance.

This invisibility has consequences. Without accurate data, we cannot quantify the burden. Without classification, we cannot guide policy. Without research, we cannot design effective treatments, and without investment, we cannot scale care.

The WHO's Intersectoral Global Action Plan (IGAP) calls on countries to strengthen information systems for neurological disorders. It asks us to identify, monitor, and track the true burden of neurological conditions across the lifespan. PCNS must be part of this effort.

We cannot afford to ignore it any longer.

Despite clear neurological symptoms, PCNS is often filed under vague labels like "post-viral fatigue" or "post COVID-19 condition." These categories are too broad. They do not help clinicians, researchers, or policymakers understand what is happening. They dilute the urgency of the problem.

In most health systems, PCNS is not separately coded. ICD-11 currently does not include a dedicated diagnosis code for PCNS. As a result, electronic health records, hospital registries, and insurance data do not capture it accurately. It is also missing from most national disease surveillance systems.

This makes it impossible to know how many people are affected. We do not know how many are referred to neurology, how many are hospitalized, how many are unemployed due to PCNS, or how many recover.

This data vacuum is dangerous. It leads to underfunding. It justifies neglect. It sends a message that this condition is not serious.

It also blocks our ability to plan care. If we can't count PCNS, we can't build services for it. We can't estimate workforce needs. We can't secure disability supports, and we can't evaluate the effectiveness of our interventions.

We must start by naming PCNS. Name it in medical records. Name it in research protocols. Name it in public health policies.

Then we must count it.

That means:

- Assigning PCNS a specific ICD code or subtype
- Embedding PCNS in electronic health record templates
- Adding PCNS to national and global neurological registries
- Developing symptom checklists and case definitions for clinical use
- Training clinicians to identify and document PCNS

Surveillance systems should be updated to capture PCNS across care settings—from primary care to neurology clinics to rehabilitation centers. This should include demographic data, clinical severity, duration, and disability status.

We should also link PCNS to mortality and long-term outcomes where relevant. Some people with PCNS experience worsening cardiovascular and neurological health over time. Tracking this is essential.

Data should be disaggregated by age, sex, socioeconomic status, and geography. We know PCNS affects women more than men. We know it is more common in frontline workers and people with limited healthcare access. Without disaggregated data, these inequities remain hidden.

4.3.5 The Role of the Global Burden of Disease (GBD) Study

One of the most important tools in global health is the Global Burden of Disease (GBD) study. It shapes global health priorities. It guides donor funding. It informs national health planning, yet PCNS is not included as a standalone neurological condition in GBD estimates. This is a critical oversight.

We urgently need GBD collaborators and health ministries to work together to include PCNS as a recognized condition in future updates. It should be measured using both prevalence and years lived with disability (YLDs). Severity distributions should reflect the profound functional impairment experienced by many patients.

We also need to model the economic impact of PCNS. How many workdays are lost? How much productivity has declined? What is the cost of delayed diagnosis and untreated symptoms?

These estimates can help make the case for national investment. They can support insurance coverage, and they can drive innovation in service delivery.

4.4 Research: A Neglected Frontier

Beyond surveillance, we need a serious research agenda. PCNS is not new anymore. We've seen millions of cases since 2020, but there is still no standardized diagnostic pathway. No approved treatments. No clear rehabilitation guidelines.

This is because PCNS research has been piecemeal and underfunded.

Most studies focus on acute COVID-19. Few follow patients for more than six months. Even fewer include neurological assessments or imaging, and most trials exclude patients with fluctuating, multisystem symptoms, the very people who need help most.

We need more than observational studies. We need trials.

We need research on:

- Neuroinflammation in PCNS
- Brain imaging findings
- Immune dysfunction and autoantibodies
- Dysautonomia mechanisms
- Cognitive rehabilitation strategies
- Longitudinal symptom tracking
- Functional recovery pathways

This research should be diverse. It should include women, ethnic minorities, rural communities, and people with disabilities. It should involve both biomedical and social sciences, and it must be designed in partnership with patients.

PCNS research must also include implementation science. How do we scale effective models of care? How do we integrate PCNS into neurology services, Long COVID clinics, and rehabilitation programs? What models work in low-resource settings?

We already have frameworks to guide this. The WHO IGAP Toolkit provides clear steps for evidence generation, stakeholder involvement, and policy translation.

But we need funding.

Governments should dedicate a percentage of COVID-19 recovery funds to PCNS research. Research agencies should prioritize calls that include neurological follow-up. Industry, philanthropic partners, and academic networks must also step up.

In Australia, we have started to build the evidence base. We have integrated PCNS into our *Life's Ten* preventive brain health campaigns. We've supported *World Brain Day* messaging focused on neurological disability prevention post-COVID.

We are working with clinics to develop screening protocols, outcome measures, and care pathways for PCNS patients. We are collaborating on data collection projects that link PCNS symptoms with biomarkers, brain imaging, and clinical outcomes.

We are calling for inclusion of PCNS in NHMRC, MRFF, and other research priorities.

But this is just the beginning. A national PCNS registry is needed. Real-world data on recovery patterns and treatment effectiveness must be collected, and international collaboration must be strengthened.

Without strong information systems, PCNS remains invisible. Without research, it remains misunderstood. Without recognition in burden of disease models, it remains underfunded. To change the story, we must measure the reality. We must name PCNS. We must count it, and we must learn from it. Only then can we deliver the care people need. Only then can we design services that work. Only then can we plan for the future. PCNS is not a mystery anymore. It is a measurable, treatable, preventable neurological syndrome. Now it's time to treat it that way.

Post-COVID-19 Neurological Syndrome (PCNS) has changed lives. Millions of people across the world now live with brain fog, fatigue, emotional dysregulation, and chronic pain. Many of them were healthy, working, and thriving before COVID-19. Today, they struggle to get out of bed, complete simple tasks, or return to work. They have lost not only their health but their sense of identity and security.

Yet, for many, the hardest part is not the symptoms, it's being ignored.

Despite the growing scientific evidence, PCNS is still not widely accepted in policy, health systems, or social support structures. The use of vague terms like "Long COVID" has created a catch-all category that dilutes the unique and disabling features of PCNS. As a result, patients are often told their condition is unclear, untreatable, or not real.

This is a failure of both science and justice.

People living with PCNS deserve recognition. They deserve access to care, and they deserve protection under human rights frameworks that ensure dignity, safety, and inclusion. The WHO's Intersectoral Global Action Plan (IGAP) on Neurological Disorders calls for inclusion of people with neurological conditions in all aspects of policy, planning, and service design. PCNS must be no exception.

4.4.1 A Health Condition That Strips Away Inclusion

Most people with PCNS do not have a formal diagnosis. Without it, they fall through the cracks. They are often denied access to disability support, workplace accommodations, or rehabilitation. Many are unemployed, not because they do not want to work, but because their symptoms make it impossible to function at full capacity.

This lack of inclusion is not only harmful, it is discriminatory.

Employment protections vary by country, but in most places, to access benefits or accommodations, a person must have a recognized diagnosis. With PCNS still missing from major classification systems like ICD-11, many patients face bureaucratic denial. They are told "You don't meet the criteria," yet they are unable to work, study, or live independently.

This legal and administrative exclusion worsens health outcomes. Financial stress, housing instability, and social isolation all contribute to further neurological and mental health decline. For people already facing stigma, the system's silence sends a clear message: you are not a priority.

This must change.

4.4.2 The Power of Lived Experience

No one understands PCNS better than those who live with it. Their voices are powerful. Their stories are evidence. Their insights can shape better research, policy, and clinical care.

That is why inclusion must be more than symbolic. People with PCNS must have a seat at every table, research committees, funding bodies, clinical guideline panels, and parliamentary hearings. They should co-design services, lead support networks, and participate in awareness campaigns.

Around the world, PCNS patients have stepped up. In Australia, the Federal Parliament's Inquiry into Long COVID and Repeated COVID Infections highlighted their stories. Testimonies from that report describe lost careers, daily cognitive struggles, emotional breakdowns, and abandonment by healthcare systems. They also show resilience, innovation, and self-advocacy in the face of systemic neglect.

These voices are not anecdotes. They are lived data. They point to patterns—failures in access, dismissal by clinicians, gaps in social policy, that no chart review can fully capture. That is why IGAP emphasizes the role of people with neurological conditions in every level of decision-making.

It is not enough to research PCNS. We must listen to it.

Stigma is one of the greatest barriers to care for people with PCNS. Because symptoms are invisible and fluctuate, patients are often disbelieved. They are told they are anxious, lazy, or imagining it. When they try to explain their condition, they are met with skepticism, even from doctors.

Part of this comes from language. The term "Long COVID" is too vague. It is associated with fatigue, not brain dysfunction. When we don't name PCNS for what it is a neurological syndrome, we reinforce the myth that it is vague or psychological.

This harms patients. It delays diagnosis. It leads to inappropriate referrals. It silences people from asking for help.

We need public education campaigns that explain what PCNS is. We need to normalize brain fog, dysautonomia, and emotional lability as real, physical outcomes of a neurological injury, and we need health professionals to be trained to recognize, validate, and manage these symptoms not dismiss them.

Reducing stigma also means protecting people with PCNS in employment, education, and social systems. Governments must enact policies that recognize episodic and fluctuating disabilities. Workplace accommodations such as flexible hours, rest breaks, and remote work must be legally supported.

Stigma thrives in silence. Naming PCNS is the first step toward breaking it.

4.4.3 Health Equity and Global Inclusion

PCNS has hit hardest in underserved populations. Many people affected are from lower socioeconomic backgrounds, marginalized communities, and countries with limited health infrastructure. The symptoms of PCNS don't respect borders, but care systems often do.

In low- and middle-income countries, neurological care was already under-resourced before the pandemic. Now, the challenge is even greater. Most of these countries have no neurologists at the primary care level. Rehabilitation services are scarce. Mental health is still stigmatized. For people with PCNS in these regions, care is simply not available.

The result? More disability. More exclusion. More economic hardship.

A human rights-based response to PCNS means building equitable systems. It means supporting telehealth, task-sharing, and community-based rehab models. It means translating information into local languages, funding travel to clinics, and providing social support to families.

Global inclusion also means including PCNS in the disability metrics of WHO, World Bank, and UN agencies. It means offering technical support to countries developing national neurological strategies under IGAP, and it means ensuring that people with PCNS in Sri Lanka, Kenya, Bolivia, or Indonesia are not left behind.

True inclusion must be global.

The first step toward protecting rights is recognition. PCNS must be recognized as a legitimate, disabling neurological condition. Once that happens, everything else becomes possible: disability benefits, legal protections, tailored care models, and global funding.

We cannot afford to wait.

The consequences of ignoring PCNS will not only be medical, they will be social, economic, and moral. If we don't act now, millions of people will remain locked out of systems designed to support them. We will fail in our duty to protect the vulnerable.

But if we do act, if we listen, name, and include, we have the chance to build something better. A health system that hears. A society that adapts. A future where brain health is not just preserved, but protected, for all.

That is what PCNS patients are asking for. Not pity, but partnership. Not sympathy, but support.

Recognition. Access. Justice. Now is the time.

Post-COVID-19 Neurological Syndrome (PCNS) has emerged as one of the most disabling and under-acknowledged consequences of the COVID-19 pandemic. As this chapter has shown, the neurological symptoms associated with PCNS are broad, sustained, and functionally devastating. They affect cognition, memory, sleep, pain regulation, emotional stability, and autonomic function. Importantly, these symptoms are not rare or mild—they are common, severe, and long-lasting for a significant portion of those affected.

Despite this, PCNS remains poorly recognized in clinical care, underrepresented in research, and almost entirely absent from national and global health policies. This disconnect between lived reality and institutional response has left millions without proper diagnosis, care, or support. This is not just a public health oversight. It is a failure of systems to adapt quickly to an evolving neurological crisis.

The WHO Intersectoral Global Action Plan (IGAP) offers a powerful and timely framework to address this gap. IGAP urges countries to integrate neurological conditions into their health systems across all stages of life. It calls for better data, workforce investment, person-centered care, public education, and protection of the rights of people with neurological disorders. PCNS fits every one of these criteria and deserves full inclusion in IGAP implementation plans globally.

This chapter has outlined how IGAP's five strategic objectives can be used to address PCNS. From integrating PCNS into national neurology strategies to developing accurate surveillance systems and promoting preventive brain health, the IGAP framework gives countries a clear roadmap for action. It does not ask nations to build new systems from scratch but to enhance and adapt what already exists. By applying IGAP to PCNS, we can strengthen care not only for this condition but for neurological health more broadly.

Prevention remains a crucial area of opportunity. The brain health movement, particularly campaigns like Life's Ten and World Brain Day, has already made significant inroads in raising awareness about the preventable aspects of neurological disability. Many PCNS risk factors—like cardiovascular instability, sleep disruption, and poor stress regulation—are modifiable. Promoting baseline brain health may reduce severity and support faster recovery among those affected.

Yet none of this progress is possible without formal recognition. PCNS must be named, coded, and tracked. It must be visible in burden of disease studies, national registries, and clinical guidelines. Only then can we build the care pathways, funding mechanisms, and research agendas required to reduce its global impact.

The stories shared by patients and supported by emerging data make the case even clearer. These are people who were working, raising children, studying, or leading organisations before COVID-19. Now, many are isolated, unemployed, or unable to function without assistance. Their symptoms are not transient inconveniences. They are neurological injuries, and they deserve a coordinated, compassionate response.

That response must also be equitable. Low- and middle-income countries face a dual challenge: a rising burden of PCNS and a shortage of neurological resources. IGAP recognises this and promotes inclusive policies that consider workforce training, task sharing, and digital health tools. PCNS care must be designed with accessibility in mind, ensuring that rural, remote, and vulnerable populations are not left behind.

Finally, none of this can succeed without partnership with the people most affected. Lived experience must be at the center of PCNS advocacy, service design, and research. These individuals are not passive patients. They are experts in what PCNS means day to day. Their insights can make systems more responsive, services more effective, and policies more humane.

PCNS is not going away. The question is whether we will rise to meet it. Will we take the lessons of IGAP and apply them? Will we build data systems that track neurological health in real time? Will we train a workforce that can recognize and treat PCNS? Will we listen to patients who are still fighting to be believed?

The tools are in front of us. The IGAP framework is ready. The challenge now is action.

4.5 Conclusion

PCNS is a global neurological crisis hiding in plain sight. It affects millions across all continents, from urban centers to rural communities. It disrupts lives, economies, and health systems, yet it remains under-recognized, mislabelled, and poorly tracked. The longer we fail to act, the more human potential is lost.

The WHO IGAP Implementation Toolkit provides an ideal structure to address this challenge. It gives countries a clear, practical, and inclusive framework to improve care for neurological conditions across the life course. By embedding PCNS into national plans, surveillance systems, care models, and workforce strategies, we can change the course of this post-pandemic burden.

More importantly, adopting IGAP principles can help prevent long-term disability, reduce stigma, and improve brain health for all. The promotion of brain health is not just a medical task. It is a social and economic imperative. A nation's brain capital is its greatest asset. When neurological health declines, so does productivity, innovation, and resilience.

Embracing the IGAP framework to respond to PCNS is about more than treating symptoms. It is about protecting futures. The cost of inaction will be measured in lost lives, lost workforces, and lost opportunities, but with the right tools, clear leadership, and a commitment to equity, we can turn the tide.

The time to act is now.

References

1. Leonardi M, Martelletti P, Burstein R, Fornari A, Grazzi L, Guekht A, et al. The World Health Organization Intersectoral Global Action Plan on Epilepsy and Other Neurological Disorders and the headache revolution: from headache burden to a global action plan for headache disorders. J Headache Pain. 2024;25(1):4.
2. Wijeratne T, Gillard Crewther S, Sales C, Karimi L. COVID-19 pathophysiology predicts that ischemic stroke occurrence is an expectation, not an exception—a systematic review. Front Neurol. 2021;11(1759):607221.
3. Wijeratne T, Crewther SG. A Systems Neuroscience Approach to Diagnosis and Rehabilitation of Post COVID Neurological Syndrome Based on the Systems Neuroscience Test Battery (SNTB) Study Protocol. NeuroRehabilitation. 2025;56(1):37–47.
4. Grisold W, Dodick DW, Guekht A, Lewis S, Wijeratne T. Brain health for all ages: a global call to action. Lancet. 2025;406(10501):329.

5. Wijeratne T, Bassetti CLA, Grisold W, Dodick D, Rouleau G, Lewis SL, et al. Brain health for all on World Brain Day 2022. Lancet Neurol. 2022;21(9):772–3.
6. Rost NS, Salinas J, Jordan JT, Banwell B, Correa DJ, Said RR, et al. The brain health imperative in the 21st century—a call to action: the AAN brain health platform and position statement. Neurology. 2023;101(13):570–9.

The Elephant We Refuse to Name: Barriers in PCNS Care

5

Reuben Parama Iswara and Tissa Wijeratne

5.1 Introduction: We Asked. They Answered. But Are We Listening?

Over the past three years, we have attended and hosted more than a dozen PCNS-focused conferences, workshops, and forums in Melbourne. Many of these were intentionally designed to be patient-centered not just conferences *about* PCNS, but conversations *with* the people who live it every day. We listened to thousands of individuals share what they've been through, what they've tried, what has failed, and what they still hope for.

What emerged was sobering and consistent. Nearly every person said the same thing in different words: *Nothing works. No one knows what's wrong. I've been passed around from doctor to doctor. And I feel completely alone.*

Despite all the published papers, webinars, rapid reviews, and emerging diagnostic models, what patients continue to experience on the ground is uncertainty, dismissal, and chaos. Many said they felt like they were losing their minds. Others said they felt invisible. Some described themselves as being caught in a maze of well-meaning clinicians, each treating one small part of a much bigger problem. They used phrases like "neurological limbo," "medical ping pong," and "a system built to miss me." [1–3]

R. Parama Iswara (✉)
Department of Neurology, Western Health, Melbourne, VIC, Australia
e-mail: Reuben.ParamaIswara@wh.org.au

T. Wijeratne
Department of Neurology and Stroke, La Trobe University, St. Albans, VIC, Australia
e-mail: tissa.wijeratne@wh.org.au

T. Wijeratne, S. Crewther (eds.), *Post Covid-19 Neurological Syndrome*,
https://doi.org/10.1007/978-3-032-14995-4_5

These are not outliers or anecdotes. These are representative voices. They span age groups, genders, professions, and levels of prior health literacy. They are speaking from lived experience and they are telling us that what we are doing is not working.

5.2 The Elephant in the Room

At every event, the same theme kept coming up. Patients described a myriad of symptoms—brain fog, unrelenting fatigue, memory lapses, emotional crashes, dizziness, heart palpitations, and sleep disturbances, and yet, even after years of advocacy, most of these individuals had no formal diagnosis.

The common phrase used was *"Long COVID,"* but patients said this didn't capture what they were experiencing. What they described matched exactly what we have detailed in earlier chapters of this book: the core features of *Post-COVID-19 Neurological Syndrome*.

But here's the problem. We are still not calling it that. Most clinicians still use vague terminology. Most hospitals do not recognize PCNS as a neurological syndrome. The scientific community continues to describe it in silos, brain fog in one study, dysautonomia in another, fatigue in yet another. It's like the old parable of the blind men and the elephant: each specialist feels one part of the animal and describes a different beast.

Until we name the full picture, we cannot treat it [4–11].

5.3 A Flood of Fragmented Solutions

In response to the growing wave of PCNS cases, clinicians and allied health professionals have tried to help, but without an agreed diagnosis, many have started building their own solutions. The result is a flood of self-published websites, untested co-designed "care pathways," and allied health protocols that often lack evidence and coherence.

Patients go from GP to physiotherapist to psychologist to naturopath, collecting fragmented advice along the way. Some try pacing apps. Others are prescribed antidepressants. Many end up spending thousands of dollars out-of-pocket, hoping that something, anything, might help.

But again and again, we hear the same story: *"I tried everything. Nothing worked. And no one really understood what was wrong."*

This is not a failure of effort. It's a failure of system design. We are asking clinicians to manage a complex neurological syndrome with no tools, no codes, no guidelines, and no institutional support. It's like asking someone to navigate a city without a map—or even a name for the place they're in.

5.4 What the Scientific Community Is Missing

The research community has published hundreds of studies on post-COVID symptoms. Many are small. Some are conflicting. Few are longitudinal, and almost none capture the full constellation of neurological, autonomic, cognitive, and emotional symptoms that patients describe.

Most studies focus on one domain fatigue, mood, heart rate variability but miss the interdependence of symptoms. Others rely on tools not designed for neurological illness: Standard depression scales, basic sleep inventories, general quality of life surveys. These are useful, but insufficient.

There is still no agreed diagnostic criteria for PCNS. No global case definition. No formal inclusion in ICD-11. No biomarker-based test, and no standard of care. This absence fuels further uncertainty. It feeds the idea that PCNS is "medically unexplained," when in fact it is medically *under-described.*

Until we define this elephant, we will continue to stumble around it, pretending it is something else.

5.5 From Listening to Action

The first step toward healing is listening, but listening alone is not enough. We must act on what we've heard.

The people who shared their stories in Melbourne did not want sympathy. They wanted validation. Direction. Accountability. A name for what they are experiencing. A care pathway that makes sense, and professionals who acknowledge that this is not just a mental health issue or a post-viral drag, it is a neurological disorder.

They also wanted systems to stop reinventing the wheel. Nearly every patient said they had filled out multiple symptom questionnaires, repeated their story dozens of times, and received a different care plan at every clinic they visited. They asked for shared records, better communication between providers, and care that is consistent, not contradictory.

This is the challenge we must address in this chapter. The barriers in PCNS care are not only clinical. They are conceptual, diagnostic, administrative, cultural, and systemic. They exist because we have refused, until now, to call this what it is, a brain-based syndrome that requires coordinated, interdisciplinary, and sustained care.

5.6 Moving Forward

This chapter will outline those barriers in detail. It will look at the diagnostic delay and confusion that patients face: The fragmentation of care, the lack of clinician training, the mismatch between patient expectations and what current services can offer, and the silence of policy systems that still do not name PCNS at all.

But we will also highlight what can be done. We will build on the WHO IGAP framework and demonstrate how naming PCNS, embedding it in health systems, and designing services around lived experience is not only possible but essential.

We have the evidence. We have the tools, and now, we have the stories.

The only question is are we ready to listen, believe, and build what people actually need?

This chapter is our answer.

5.7 Understanding the Elephant: Why We Must Do Better Research—With, Not Just on, Patients

If there's one message we've heard again and again from people living with PCNS, it's this *"I feel like no one is really trying to figure this out."* Not seriously, not urgently, and certainly not with the full picture in mind.

This is the core of our problem. We are attempting to describe a complex, disabling, multisystem neurological syndrome using siloed thinking and isolated studies. It is like examining one leg of an elephant and deciding it is a tree, or touching the tail and calling it a rope. Every researcher is describing a piece of PCNS, but few are seeing the whole.

We will never understand PCNS through fragmented efforts. We need cohesive, collaborative, large-scale, and patient-informed research, starting now.

5.8 A Fractured Landscape

Right now, the global PCNS research landscape is scattered. There are hundreds of small observational studies looking at fatigue, cognition, sleep, or heart rate variability. A few clinical trials are testing single interventions. Some groups are running neuroimaging studies. Others are building small registries. Many of these projects are isolated, underpowered, and uncoordinated.

Worse, many do not involve people with lived experience in any meaningful way.

This has led to a research culture where the same questions are asked again and again, but the insights rarely translate into clinical practice. Patients are often left out of the design phase. Their voices are included at the end, if at all. This is not just inefficient—it's disrespectful.

People with PCNS are the real-world experts. They know what it feels like to crash after a short walk, to forget the names of their children, and to fear that they are losing their minds. We must invite them into the center of the research process, not as subjects—but as partners.

5.9 From Participants to Partners

Genuine co-design is not a box-ticking exercise. It means involving patients from the start: Asking what questions matter to them, letting them shape how symptoms are measured, including them in interpreting findings, sharing results in language they can understand, and most importantly, closing the loop between research and care.

Some projects are starting to do this. In Melbourne, we've begun integrating patient voices into grant writing and study design. We've asked people with PCNS what matters to them—what outcomes they care about, what interventions are worth trying, and how we can make the research process more transparent and respectful.

The feedback has been clear. People want to know:

- What is happening in their brains?
- Why do their symptoms fluctuate?
- What is the long-term trajectory?
- What can they do to feel better today, not in five years?

These are not trivial questions. They are clinical questions, research questions, and human questions. They deserve answers.

5.10 We Need Large, Multidisciplinary Cohorts

PCNS is too complex to be understood through small, single-domain studies. We need longitudinal, multidisciplinary cohorts that follow patients over time and assess a wide range of symptoms, systems, and outcomes. These studies must include brain imaging, blood-based biomarkers, cognitive testing, autonomic function, and mental health assessments—all in one place.

We also need to map these findings to real-life function: work capacity, social participation, fatigue levels, sleep quality, and mobility, and we must stratify the data by age, gender, geography, and comorbidity. Only then can we begin to understand the subtypes of PCNS—and which interventions work best for whom.

There is precedent for this. We've built national stroke registries, dementia biobanks, and cancer cohorts. We can do the same for PCNS, but only if we stop pretending this is a short-term or fringe issue.

PCNS must be recognized as a research priority in every country. It must be included in government funding calls. Institutions should support multidisciplinary PCNS research centres. Journals must publish high-quality, patient-led work—not just reviews and repackaged datasets.

Right now, many clinicians and researchers are developing their own tools to assess PCNS symptoms: New questionnaires, new fatigue scales, new apps. Each one different from the next.

This innovation is well-intentioned, but chaotic. It makes it difficult to compare results across studies. It confuses clinicians and frustrates patients. We need to agree on core outcome sets for PCNS research, validated, sensitive, and relevant.

The WHO's IGAP toolkit calls for standardized data collection and shared indicators. We should apply this to PCNS immediately. What symptoms should be tracked? What constitutes recovery? How do we define meaningful improvement? Let's decide together—with patients in the room.

We also need shared data platforms: Registries that talk to each other, and systems that protect privacy but allow collaboration. Only then can we accelerate discovery and reduce duplication.

5.11 Research Must Lead to Change

At every Melbourne forum, patients asked *"What will come from all this data collection?"* It's a fair question.

For too long, people have been asked to fill out symptom surveys, join waiting lists, and donate time and energy they barely have. In return, they get little more than a thank-you. This must change.

Research into PCNS must be linked to care. If a patient scores high for orthostatic intolerance, they should be referred for POTS assessment. If they show cognitive decline, they should be offered neurorehabilitation. Studies should offer referrals, not just results. Feedback, not just follow-up.

We must close the gap between research and real-world benefit, and we must publish results in ways that communities can understand and use.

5.12 We Need Urgency and Accountability

PCNS is not just a medical mystery. It is a growing social and economic crisis. Millions of people are out of work. Families are under strain. Health systems are overwhelmed, yet governments still treat PCNS as a vague, emerging issue, not the full-scale neurological emergency that it is.

We must act with urgency. This includes fast-tracking funding, removing red tape from ethics approvals, supporting early-career researchers, and embedding PCNS into every neurological research network.

We must also track progress. How many studies include patient partners? How many use the term PCNS? How many trials are measuring function, not just symptom scores?

Let's measure what matters, and let's hold ourselves accountable.

5.13 Care Fragmentation: Why the Health System Fails to Hold the Whole Patient

One of the most striking themes to emerge from patient stories, especially at the Melbourne forums, is how broken and disconnected the current healthcare response is to PCNS. Most patients we heard from have seen multiple doctors. Many have been referred to specialists. Neurology, cardiology, psychiatry, immunology, and more, only to find that no one clinician sees the full picture. Each one manages a symptom or two. None are responsible for the whole.

This is care fragmentation in its most painful form. Not only is it inefficient. It is harmful. Patients feel like they are being passed around. They fill out the same forms, repeat their story again and again, and still leave appointments with no answers. One patient said, "It's like being thrown between departments in a hospital where no one has read your chart." Another described it more bluntly: "I'm the glue holding my care together and I'm falling apart."

The underlying issue is structural. PCNS is a multisystem neurological syndrome. It does not fit neatly into one specialty. Its symptoms span brain, heart, lungs, gut, and mood, but our health systems are not designed to treat overlapping conditions across multiple body systems. They are built on silos, and silos do not serve people with PCNS.

A neurologist may assess cognitive symptoms but ignore gut issues. A cardiologist may treat tachycardia but dismiss fatigue. A psychologist may focus on mood but miss signs of dysautonomia. This narrow lens fails the patient every time, and because most PCNS patients have normal basic tests, they are often left in diagnostic limbo, too sick to ignore, too "undiagnosable" to treat.

Even where integrated clinics exist, care is often still not truly connected. A single multidisciplinary appointment may bring together a few professionals, but without shared goals, joint decision-making, or a long-term care plan, the outcome remains piecemeal. True integration means more than co-location. It means coordination, continuity, and accountability.

This fragmentation also shows up in communication. Many patients report that their providers do not speak to one another. Specialists send letters to GPs with vague conclusions. Allied health teams operate independently. There is no central case manager or coordinator. As a result, critical pieces of information get lost. Treatments contradict each other. Medications are prescribed without full knowledge of what else the patient is taking.

In some systems, the burden falls on the general practitioner, but most GPs are overwhelmed, undertrained in post-viral neurology, and not resourced to manage long-term neurological disability. Without clear guidelines or pathways, they do their best—but many simply do not have the tools.

Patients are then left to self-manage a complex condition that even specialists do not fully understand. They track their symptoms, chase referrals, research online, and try to piece together their own recovery plans. It is exhausting, and for many, it is unsustainable.

This problem is not unique to Australia. Around the world, people with PCNS report similar experiences. In the UK, patients describe "ping-ponging" between Long COVID clinics and their GP. In the USA, care depends heavily on private insurance coverage and varies wildly by state. In low- and middle-income countries, where specialist care is already scarce, many have no access to PCNS-informed care at all.

The consequences are far-reaching: Delayed diagnosis, inappropriate treatment, worsening disability, lost productivity, mental health decline, social isolation, caregiver burden, and mounting costs to the healthcare system with very little to show for it.

This kind of care failure would be unacceptable for other neurological conditions. We would never manage Parkinson's disease or multiple sclerosis with uncoordinated referrals and a rotating cast of one-off appointments. Why are we tolerating it for PCNS?

Part of the problem is that PCNS still lacks formal recognition. Without a diagnostic code or agreed care model, health systems do not know where to place it. There is no pathway, no funding line, and often no champion within the system. So, patients fall through the cracks. They are told to wait, to try pacing, and to come back if things get worse.

This is not care. It is abandonment.

The irony is that many of the components needed for good PCNS care already exist. Neurologists understand cognitive dysfunction. Physiotherapists can guide pacing and energy conservation. Psychologists can support adjustment and resilience. Cardiologists can assess autonomic instability. Occupational therapists can help with returning to work or study, but these resources are not aligned. They are not joined by a central framework.

What we need is an integrated care model—one that starts with recognition and ends with recovery support. This model must be built on core principles: a named diagnosis, a shared understanding of symptoms, a central care coordinator, and a flexible, person-centred plan.

Every patient with PCNS should have access to a multidisciplinary team that meets regularly, shares notes, tracks progress, and adjusts treatment over time. Care plans should include input from the patient, reflect their goals, and be updated as symptoms evolve. There should be clear lines of communication between hospital, community, and primary care settings.

Such a model does not need to be expensive. In fact, better coordination would reduce unnecessary tests, redundant referrals, and harmful treatment delays. It would also help identify those at risk of deterioration earlier, saving hospital beds and emergency visits.

Some countries have already piloted variations of this. The UK's Post-COVID Assessment Clinics aimed to bring multiple specialties together. In Canada, community health centres have adapted chronic disease management frameworks for Long COVID. In Australia, some GP-led models are experimenting with digital case conferencing and shared care planning. These are steps in the right direction.

But to scale them, we need leadership, investment, and national commitment, and we need to give these models a neurological backbone, by officially recognising PCNS for what it is.

We also need to support patients outside the clinic. Care does not stop at discharge. Many people need home-based rehab, online support groups, workplace accommodations, and disability advocacy. A truly integrated approach extends beyond medicine and includes social services, education, and public health.

At its core, PCNS care must be designed around people, not systems. That means listening to what patients actually need. Making the system work for them, and not asking them to chase fragmented pieces of a care puzzle we ourselves refuse to complete.

5.14 Discussion

Post-COVID-19 Neurological Syndrome (PCNS) is one of the most pressing yet poorly addressed health issues of our time. As shown throughout this chapter, the barriers to effective care are not subtle—they are structural, cultural, and conceptual. Despite widespread symptoms and lived experience that clearly point to brain-based dysfunction, the global response remains fragmented and insufficient.

What patients are describing is not rare. It is not vague. It is not beyond our scientific understanding. It is a multisystem neurological disorder that we have so far failed to name, study, or treat in a coordinated way. At every Melbourne forum, in every patient story, one message has come through with striking clarity: the current system does not see the whole person. Clinicians manage parts. Systems track nothing. Research describes slices of the syndrome but rarely the full elephant.

The problem begins with diagnostic ambiguity. Without a clearly accepted term like PCNS, many health systems continue to use broad labels such as "Long COVID" or "post-viral fatigue." These may capture general distress but do not describe what is truly going on. Brain fog, dysautonomia, cognitive impairment, emotional instability, and central fatigue are not psychological symptoms—they are neurological. They demand neurological attention, yet without formal diagnostic codes, PCNS remains invisible in health records, insurance systems, and research registries.

This invisibility leads to a cascade of care failures. Patients are passed between specialties. No one takes ownership. No one builds a long-term plan. Patients are left to act as their own case managers, despite being exhausted and overwhelmed. GPs are expected to coordinate, but they are not trained or resourced to manage such complex neurological recovery. Even in high-resource settings, care is fragmented and frustrating. In lower-resource regions, care is simply unavailable.

Equally alarming is the lack of meaningful research coordination. Across the world, small pilot studies, disconnected registries, and self-directed protocols abound—but few efforts look at the whole. Funding remains minimal. Data is scattered. Many researchers continue to describe parts of PCNS while ignoring the syndrome as a whole. This kind of fragmentation leads to duplication, wasted resources, and stalled progress.

We must now stop asking whether PCNS is real. We must ask why we are still acting like it isn't.

The IGAP framework provides a way forward. Its five strategic pillars. Governance, service delivery, promotion and prevention, research and information systems, and human rights—map directly onto the barriers we see in PCNS care. The framework does not ask health systems to create something entirely new. It asks them to strengthen what already exists, fill gaps, and commit to inclusion.

We already have neurology services. Let us adapt them to support PCNS care. We already have training frameworks. Let us add PCNS education. We already have disability laws. Let us ensure they apply to PCNS. We already run public campaigns about stroke, dementia, and epilepsy. Let us now talk openly about post-viral neurological syndromes too.

We also have a strong foundation in lived experience advocacy. The patients who came to our conferences, the people who filled out our surveys, the families who reached out to share their stories. They are not just waiting for change. They are building it. What they need is to be included, supported, and heard.

To truly change the PCNS care landscape, we must:

- Adopt the term PCNS globally and embed it into diagnostic systems.
- Develop coordinated, interdisciplinary care pathways with shared records.
- Create national registries and integrate PCNS into existing neurological datasets.
- Fund multidisciplinary, longitudinal research at scale.
- Include people with lived experience in the design of all studies and services.
- Train primary and specialist care providers to identify and manage PCNS.
- Use the IGAP toolkit to align local, national, and global responses.

These steps are not just about building better care—they are about restoring trust. Every time a patient is dismissed or misdiagnosed, we erode that trust. Every time a clinician says "we don't know what to do," we reinforce despair, but when we name the problem, fund its solution, and treat the person—not just the symptom—we begin to rebuild that trust.

This is not an impossible task. It is already happening in small ways. Clinics are forming. Education sessions are being run. Some systems are trialling integrated care models, but we must move from isolated pilots to system-wide reform. The scale of the problem demands it.

PCNS is not the first condition to challenge modern healthcare. HIV, ME/CFS, fibromyalgia, and traumatic brain injury were all once misunderstood and minimised. Over time, we developed language, research, and policy frameworks that helped us respond more effectively. We can—and must—do the same for PCNS.

5.15 Conclusion

Post-COVID-19 Neurological Syndrome has been described as the hidden pandemic within a pandemic. It affects millions of people worldwide. It touches every continent, every age group, and every healthcare system, and yet, we continue to ignore it, delay it, or downplay it.

This chapter has argued that the greatest barrier to PCNS care is not a lack of treatments. It is a lack of recognition. Until we name the condition, we cannot track it. Until we track it, we cannot build care systems, and until we build care systems, patients will continue to suffer in silence.

The WHO IGAP Implementation Toolkit gives us the blueprint we need. It shows us how to integrate neurological care into public health policy, how to build coordinated services, how to strengthen research and data collection, and how to uphold the rights of people with neurological conditions. If we apply IGAP to PCNS, we not only improve care for this group, we strengthen brain health across the life course for all people [12–15].

Brain health is not a niche issue. It is central to national well-being. When brain function is compromised, so is education, work, parenting, and creativity. When we neglect neurological conditions like PCNS, we are not just creating disability we are undermining our collective brain capital.

If we fail to act, the cost will be enormous. Health systems will face increasing demand. Economies will lose productive citizens. Trust in medicine will erode, but if we embrace IGAP, include patients as partners, and make PCNS a national and global priority, we can create meaningful change.

The elephant is not going away, but we can stop pretending it isn't there.

Now is the time to call it by its name. Post-COVID-19 Neurological Syndrome. Let's start building systems worthy of the people it affects.

References

1. Donnelly SC. After acute there is the long-COVID syndrome: what's the plan? QJM. 2022;115(1):1–2.
2. Quinn KL, Razak F, Cheung AM. Assessing common and potentially modifiable symptoms of post-COVID-19 condition (long COVID) in adults. CMAJ. 2023;195(2):E76–e7.
3. Fowler-Davis S, Young R, Maden-Wilkinson T, Hameed W, Dracas E, Hurrell E, et al. Assessing the acceptability of a co-produced long COVID intervention in an underserved community in the UK. Int J Environ Res Public Health. 2021;18(24):13191.
4. Singh B, Kaur P, Maroules M. Autoimmune hepatitis-primary biliary cholangitis overlap syndrome triggered by COVID-19. Eur J Case Rep Intern Med. 2021;8(3):002264.
5. Lv Y, Zhang T, Cai J, Huang C, Zhan S, Liu J. Bioinformatics and systems biology approach to identify the pathogenetic link of long COVID and Myalgic encephalomyelitis/chronic fatigue syndrome. Front Immunol. 2022;13:952987.
6. Lai Y-J, Liu S-H, Manachevakul S, Lee T-A, Kuo C-T, Bello D. Biomarkers in long COVID-19: a systematic review. Front Med. 2023;10:10.

7. Wijeratne T, Wijeratne C. Clinical utility of serial systemic immune inflammation indices (SSIIi) in the context of post covid-19 neurological syndrome (PCNS). J Neurol Sci. 2021;423:117356.
8. Wijeratne T, Gillard Crewther S, Sales C, Karimi L. COVID-19 pathophysiology predicts that ischemic stroke occurrence is an expectation, not an exception-a systematic review. Front Neurol. 2020;11:607221.
9. Wijeratne T, Gillard Crewther S, Sales C, Karimi L. COVID-19 pathophysiology predicts that ischemic stroke occurrence is an expectation, not an exception—a systematic review. Front Neurol. 2021;11:1759.
10. Wijeratne T, Crewther S. Post-COVID 19 neurological syndrome (PCNS); a novel syndrome with challenges for the global neurology community. J Neurol Sci. 2020;419:117179.
11. Wijeratne T, Crewther SG. A systems neuroscience approach to diagnosis and rehabilitation of post COVID neurological syndrome based on the systems neuroscience test battery (SNTB) study protocol. NeuroRehabilitation. 2025;56(1):37–47.
12. Chatys-Bogacka Z, Mazurkiewicz I, Slowik J, Bociaga-Jasik M, Dzieza-Grudnik A, Slowik A, et al. Brain fog and quality of life at work in non-hospitalized patients after COVID-19. Int J Environ Res Public Health. 2022;19(19).
13. Grisold W, Dodick DW, Guekht A, Lewis S, Wijeratne T. Brain health for all ages: a global call to action. Lancet. 2025;406(10501):329.
14. Wijeratne T, Bassetti CLA, Grisold W, Dodick D, Rouleau G, Lewis SL, et al. Brain health for all on world brain day 2022. Lancet Neurol. 2022;21(9):772–3.
15. Rost NS, Salinas J, Jordan JT, Banwell B, Correa DJ, Said RR, et al. The brain health imperative in the 21st century-a call to action: the AAN brain health platform and position statement. Neurology. 2023;101(13):570–9.

6 A Call for Services: Building the System PCNS Patients Deserve

Shanika Nandasiri and Tissa Wijeratne

6.1 Introduction: We Must Build Together Services, Education, and Research, with Patients at the Center

The COVID-19 pandemic has changed the world [1], but for millions, it did not end when the virus left their body [2–12]. They are living with a new condition, a persistent condition, a disabling neurological syndrome we now call Post COVID-19 Neurological Syndrome, or PCNS.

These individuals are not rare. They are everywhere. They are teachers who cannot read a page without forgetting what it said. Parents who struggle to get out of bed. Nurses who once ran wards but now rely on others for help. Young people who cannot finish a degree. Older adults who feel they are losing themselves.

At community forums in Melbourne and around the world, we have heard their stories. Over and over again. People say the same things. "Nothing works." "No one understands what is happening to me." "Every doctor gives me a different answer." "I am scared that I will never recover." These voices deserve more than sympathy. They deserve a system that responds with urgency, intelligence, and compassion.

That system must rest on three strong foundations: Services, Education, Research. Without all three, our response will continue to fall short, but these pillars cannot stand alone. They must be built together, and they must be built with patients and families at the center.

We cannot continue to build around them. We must walk with them.

S. Nandasiri (✉)
Western Health, Melbourne, VIC, Australia
e-mail: Shanika.Nandasiri@wh.org.au

T. Wijeratne
Department of Neurology and Stroke, La Trobe University, St. Albans, VIC, Australia
e-mail: tissa.wijeratne@wh.org.au

T. Wijeratne, S. Crewther (eds.), *Post Covid-19 Neurological Syndrome*,
https://doi.org/10.1007/978-3-032-14995-4_6

6.2 Services

Most people with PCNS do not receive care that fits their needs [5–7]. Many do not receive any care at all. They are passed between specialists, sent home with no plan, given advice that does not help, or worse, advice that harms.

This is not because health workers do not care. It is because the system does not know what to do. There is no agreed pathway, no central clinic in most areas, no care coordinator, no standard follow-up, and no roadmap.

What we need is not a miracle. It is a structured and coordinated care response. One that recognizes PCNS as a real neurological condition. One that brings together primary care, neurology, rehabilitation, mental health, and allied health. One that is flexible enough to work in hospitals and community settings, in person and online, rural and urban.

The services we need already exist, but they are scattered, disconnected, and often hard to access. We must bring them together under one name, one model, one mission.

6.3 Education

Too many health professionals have never heard of PCNS [12, 13], or they do not know what it looks like, or they dismiss it as anxiety, burnout, or tiredness. This is not their fault. PCNS is new, but the impact of this knowledge gap is profound.

Patients are left feeling unheard. Unseen. Misdiagnosed. They are told to "push through." They are given antidepressants when they need autonomic testing, or told to exercise when they need to rest.

Education can change this, not just in hospitals, but in medical schools, in nursing schools, physiotherapy programs, and GP training. We need simple tools that help people recognize PCNS early, know when to refer, know what to say, and know what not to say.

Education must go further. Employers need to know how to support staff. Schools need to understand how to help children with brain fog. Families need guidance, and the general public needs to know this is not made up. It is real. It is physical. It is neurological.

Knowledge is not enough unless it leads to empathy. Our education must be clinical, but also deeply human.

6.4 Research

We cannot solve what we do not study. PCNS is still poorly understood. We do not yet know why some people develop it, or why others recover quickly. We do not know which treatments work best. We do not know how long symptoms will last, or how to predict recovery.

Most research so far has been small, scattered, focused on one symptom at a time: Fatigue in one paper, brain fog in another, dizziness in the next. This is like looking at pieces of a puzzle without ever putting them together.

We need real investment, in large studies that follow people over time, look at blood markers, brain scans, cognitive testing, functional recovery. We need clinical trials not just observation: Trials of rehabilitation, trials of pacing, trials of medication, trials of combined treatments not quick fixes, but thoughtful, patient-informed science.

And we need research that is not just about patients, but with patients, designed by them, guided by their goals, interpreted through their experience. Patients are the experts in living with this condition. We must learn from them.

6.5 Walking with Patients and Families

PCNS does not affect one person. It affects entire families. Partners become carers. Parents become advocates. Children take on roles they are too young for. These families need support too.

We must stop asking patients to navigate this alone. We must walk beside them, from diagnosis, to recovery, and beyond. That means designing services with them, creating education materials that reflect their voice, shaping research questions around their lives.

This is not just about what we do. It is how we do it. It means listening without rushing, explaining without blame, offering hope without false promises, giving practical help, but also acknowledging the loss, the grief, the fear.

It means treating people as people not puzzles.

6.6 The Time Is Now

We cannot delay. Every week more people join this group. More leave their jobs, drop out of school, lose their independence, their identity, their voice. Every day we delay is a day of preventable suffering.

We know how to build these pillars: Services, Education, Research. We have done it before, for stroke, epilepsy, brain injury. Now we must do it for PCNS.

What we need is focus, funding, leadership, and most of all, will.

Let us not wait until the burden becomes overwhelming. Let us act now, with patients, with families, with courage. PCNS is real. The need is urgent, and the path is clear. Let us walk it, together.

6.7 Building the First Pillar: Services that Truly Support People with PCNS

We cannot treat what we do not name, and we cannot heal what we do not serve. At present, people with Post COVID-19 Neurological Syndrome face a gaping hole in healthcare systems. They live with a disabling condition, yet they are left without coordinated care, without diagnostic certainty, without any roadmap. The first step in responding to this crisis is to build services that reflect the true nature of PCNS, services that listen, services that integrate, and services that actually work.

At the core of this effort is one truth. PCNS is not a simple condition. It is not limited to one part of the body or one medical specialty. It affects cognition, sleep, fatigue, emotion, pain regulation, and the autonomic nervous system. It affects work, learning, parenting, and social function. This is not a single-symptom illness. It is a full-body experience rooted in the brain.

That is why PCNS cannot be managed by a single provider, or even a single clinic. We need a new kind of service model. One that brings disciplines together. One that is led by the needs of the patient, and one that is flexible enough to adapt as symptoms shift and evolve.

6.8 What Does a PCNS Service Look Like

A good PCNS service starts with recognition. The patient is seen, heard, taken seriously. They are given time. Their full symptom picture is recorded. Their history is not rushed or dismissed. From there, the service builds a coordinated plan, not one specialist at a time, but a team approach: A neurologist, a general practitioner, a rehabilitation physician, a psychologist, a physiotherapist, a sleep specialist, and if needed, a social worker or occupational therapist.

Each team member brings a piece of the puzzle, but they work together. They meet regularly. They communicate. They use shared notes. They align around one set of goals. This is not a scattered referral chain. It is a unified model of care.

The service does not end at diagnosis. It continues through recovery. It adapts. If brain fog worsens, cognitive rehabilitation is adjusted. If new autonomic symptoms appear, testing is arranged. If fatigue becomes unmanageable, the pacing plan is updated. The team walks with the patient, not ahead, not behind, but beside.

6.9 Key Features of Effective PCNS Services

There are several principles that must guide PCNS service design. First, accessibility. Services must be available to rural and regional communities, that means telehealth, local coordination, and mobile teams where possible. Second, affordability. Care must not be limited to those who can pay. PCNS services must be part of universal coverage or publicly funded programs.

Third, flexibility. PCNS does not follow a single timeline. Some recover in months. Others take years. Services must be designed for long-term engagement with regular reviews not just one-off assessments. Fourth, personalization. No two cases of PCNS are identical. Care plans must reflect the individual's goals, challenges, and context.

Fifth, communication. Patients must understand what is happening. They must be given clear explanations, written summaries, and contacts for follow-up. They must not feel like they are navigating blind.

And finally, integration. PCNS care must link into existing neurological services, but also into mental health care, pain clinics, disability support, and employment services. It must bridge the gap between hospital and home.

6.10 Learning from Other Conditions

We do not have to invent this model from scratch. We have examples to learn from. Stroke care has evolved from fragmented to coordinated with stroke units, shared protocols, rehab pathways, case managers, and multidisciplinary meetings. We must do the same for PCNS.

Multiple sclerosis services offer another model. Patients are followed over time. Their needs are reassessed. Services are flexible. Teams work together, and the condition is accepted as real and deserving of long-term support.

The key difference is that those conditions are already classified, recognized, funded. PCNS is not, but it can be, and it must be.

6.11 Why It Matters

Without services, patients fall through cracks. They end up in emergency departments when symptoms crash. They are given tests that show nothing. They are sent home feeling hopeless. They are told to wait, to rest, to manage on their own.

This leads to worsening disability, social isolation, mental health decline, lost jobs, strained families, and in many cases, preventable harm. We must change the system before more lives are derailed.

Providing coordinated care is not just an ethical responsibility. It is economically wise. Supporting recovery reduces long-term cost. It keeps people in the workforce. It prevents dependence. It builds resilience. The return on investment is clear.

6.12 What Patients Are Telling Us

Patients with PCNS are not passive. They are experts in their own condition. They want to be part of the care process, but they need to be guided not abandoned.

They tell us they want one place to go, one team to talk to. They want answers, but even more, they want continuity. They are tired of repeating their story, of being told conflicting things, of being bounced between departments.

They want help with returning to work, managing daily life, explaining their condition to others. They want options for rehab, for therapy, for recovery.

And above all, they want to be believed.

6.13 Moving Forward

We must build these services now. Health departments should fund pilot PCNS clinics. Hospitals should adapt existing neurorehabilitation teams. Medical colleges should publish care guidelines. National bodies should develop care pathways.

These services should be evaluated, patient outcomes tracked, lessons shared, models refined, then scaled.

This is the first step in a much bigger journey, but it is the one that matters most. Because without care, all the education and research in the world will not ease suffering.

We have waited long enough. Patients have waited too long. Let us build the care they deserve.

Building the Second Pillar: Education that Changes Minds and Systems.

The care gap for people living with Post COVID-19 Neurological Syndrome does not exist only because of a lack of services. It also exists because of a profound lack of understanding. Too many health professionals still do not know how to recognize PCNS. Too many still believe it is stress, anxiety, or burnout. Patients are told to rest, to wait it out, to think positive, and sometimes, to stop talking about it altogether.

This is not due to malice. It is due to a lack of training. PCNS is not yet a formal part of most medical curricula. It does not appear in the textbooks. It is not included in standard lectures. Most junior doctors and nurses have never seen a structured approach to PCNS, and even seasoned clinicians may never have encountered a clear protocol for how to support someone experiencing brain fog, dysautonomia, or post-exertional crashes.

This is why education is the second essential pillar in our response to PCNS. Without better knowledge, we will not achieve better care. Without better training, even the best services will fail, and without better understanding, the stigma will only grow.

6.14 Training Clinicians at Every Level

PCNS is not limited to neurology clinics. Most patients first seek help in general practice, or in emergency departments, or with a physiotherapist, or a mental health professional. That means education must reach every part of the system.

General practitioners need to be trained to screen for common PCNS symptoms. They need tools to identify when someone needs referral to neurology or rehabilitation. They need guidance on managing energy levels, sleep disruption, and cognitive problems.

Specialists in neurology, cardiology, psychiatry, and rehabilitation also need more targeted training. Many of them still work with outdated models of post-viral recovery. Many are still unfamiliar with how to assess autonomic instability or neuroinflammatory symptoms without structural lesions on scans.

Allied health professionals play a vital role in PCNS care. Physiotherapists need to be educated about pacing and post-exertional symptom exacerbation. Occupational therapists should be equipped to support cognitive retraining and return-to-work planning. Psychologists need to understand the neurobiological drivers of emotional dysregulation and cognitive dysfunction.

This education must be practical. It must be case-based. It should be delivered in accessible formats: Short videos, webinars, clinical tip sheets, interactive modules, and it must be endorsed by credible national and international bodies. When professional colleges and associations take the lead, clinicians listen.

6.15 Medical and Allied Health Curricula

To change the future, we must teach the next generation. PCNS should be included in medical school teaching, nursing curricula, physiotherapy training programs, psychology placements, and public health degrees. Students must learn how to ask the right questions, how to look beyond normal tests, how to validate symptoms, and how to listen carefully.

More importantly, they must learn that post-viral neurological conditions are not new, and they are not rare. PCNS may be the most visible now, but others exist: From ME/CFS to post-dengue syndromes to neurological Lyme disease. We must teach syndromic thinking, clinical humility, and person-centered care.

Curriculum reform is not a small task, but PCNS has shown us that we cannot afford to keep training clinicians without equipping them for what is actually walking through their clinic doors. Thousands of patients later, the message is clear. What we are doing is not enough.

6.16 Educating the Public

The education gap does not stop at clinicians. The public also needs to understand what PCNS is. At present, most people still see it as a vague form of Long COVID. They do not know how disabling it can be. They do not understand why someone who looks healthy may still be unable to think clearly, or why someone who ran marathons now struggles to walk to the mailbox.

We need public awareness campaigns. These should focus on real stories, clear information, and reducing blame. They should be built in partnership with patient advocates shared through health departments, local councils, employers, schools, and media outlets.

Social media is an important tool. So are community radio stations, school newsletters, and workplace education programs. The message must be simple. PCNS is real. It is brain-based. It is common, and it is treatable, but only when recognized early and supported properly.

Public understanding is also essential for supporting return-to-work planning. Many patients feel pressure to recover faster than they can. Some lose their jobs. Others are accused of exaggeration. Education can shift workplace culture. Help employers offer realistic accommodations, and empower people to ask for what they need.

6.17 Supporting Families and Carers

Education also matters for the people closest to those with PCNS: Family members, partners, parents, friends. They are often the first to notice changes, but they may not understand what is happening. They may think their loved one is just tired, anxious, or lacking motivation.

This can create tension, frustration, even broken relationships. Families need support too: Written guides, Videos, Online workshops, Counselling, Peer groups. They need to understand that this condition is not a character flaw. It is neurological, and it is hard.

They also need practical tools: How to pace daily activities, How to help someone manage sensory overload, How to navigate appointments, How to access services. The more we support families, the more we support the patient.

6.18 Learning from the Patients Themselves

Perhaps the most important teachers of all are the patients. They have lived through this. They have tried every medication, every pacing method, every clinic, every suggestion. Their insight is profound. We must stop treating them as passive recipients of care. They are our educators, our guides.

Patients should help lead education sessions, co-author training materials, review health literacy resources, speak to student groups, share what works, and what does not.

In Melbourne, we have already seen the power of patient educators. They speak with clarity, with grace, and with truth. Their lived experience adds depth that no lecture can replace.

6.19 From Knowledge to Action

Education alone is not the answer, but without it, nothing else works. We cannot deliver good services without trained staff. We cannot build research agendas without informed questions, and we cannot create just systems if the people within them do not understand what PCNS actually is.

This is the moment to act not next year, not after more trials, but now. We know enough to teach the basics. We know enough to train for compassion, and we know that learning must go both ways.

Let us educate not just to inform, but to transform.

6.20 Building the Third Pillar: Research that Leads to Real Solutions

The lack of coordinated research into Post COVID-19 Neurological Syndrome is not just a scientific oversight. It is a humanitarian failure. Patients across the world are describing the same patterns: Brain fog, Fatigue, Headache, Autonomic instability, Mood and sleep disruption. These are not vague symptoms. They are signs of a serious and widespread neurological condition.

And yet, most national and international research systems have not prioritized this condition. In some countries, PCNS is still described as a "potential post-viral concern." In others, it is buried inside broader Long COVID studies with little attention to its neurological core. What we need now is not more surveys or commentaries. We need real research, research that is comprehensive, research that is inclusive, and research that makes a difference in patients' lives.

6.21 The Case for Research Urgency

PCNS is disabling people during their most productive years. These are not end-of-life conditions. They affect students, parents, nurses, engineers, teachers, artists, and carers. Many were previously healthy and fully independent. Now they struggle to hold jobs or complete basic daily tasks. The long-term social and economic impact of this condition is enormous.

We do not yet know how long symptoms will last. We do not know how many will fully recover. We do not know what treatments work best. These are urgent questions, and every month we wait is a missed opportunity to improve lives and reduce suffering.

6.22 What Kind of Research Do We Need

First, we need large-scale longitudinal studies. We must follow people over time, months, and years. We need to document how symptoms change, what patterns emerge, who improves, and who deteriorates. We need to track cognitive function, sleep quality, autonomic function, emotional health, and work participation over time.

Second, we need biobanking. We must collect and analyze blood, cerebrospinal fluid, saliva, and other tissues to identify biomarkers. We must look for inflammatory markers: Autoantibodies, Viral fragments, Genetic susceptibilities. This kind of research can help us develop diagnostic tests, and move us away from subjective diagnosis alone.

Third, we need brain imaging, Functional MRI, PET scans, and advanced neuroimaging protocols. These can help us see what is happening in the brain during and after infection. They can help us understand the structural and functional basis for brain fog and emotional dysregulation.

Fourth, we need clinical trials. Observational research is not enough. We must test therapies: Pharmacologic, Behavioural, Nutritional, Neuromodulatory, Integrative. We must study rehabilitation programs: Cognitive retraining, Graded activity pacing, Psychological support models, and we must do this with rigour.

Fifth, we need health systems research. How do people access care? What are the barriers? How does cost affect outcomes? What models of service delivery work best? Which ones reduce disability? Which ones increase trust and continuity? These questions are just as important as biological ones.

Finally, we need social and qualitative research. We must understand the lived experience: The grief, the loss, the resilience. We must document what patients face at home, in the workplace, and in clinics. This type of data helps policymakers and planners design systems that truly meet real needs.

6.23 Research Must Be Patient-Led

Too much research in the early pandemic was designed without patients in the room. That cannot happen now. PCNS research must be built with patients not around them, not about them, but with them.

That means involving patients in every step: Designing the research questions, Reviewing the protocols, Interpreting the data, Sharing the findings. Research must reflect the reality of the people it serves, not only what is convenient to study in a lab.

Patients can tell us what outcomes matter. It is not only about symptom scales. It is about function: Energy, Independence, Quality of life, Feeling heard, Getting back to the life they want. These are the real outcomes of interest, and they must shape what we measure and report.

We also need to ensure that research includes diverse populations. Many PCNS studies so far have focused on middle-class patients in high-income countries, but

PCNS affects everyone, across age, income, race, region, culture, language. We need inclusive recruitment, community partnerships, and cultural safety.

6.24 Funding and Coordination

None of this is possible without funding. Governments must dedicate part of their COVID-19 research budgets to PCNS. Research councils must issue specific calls. Philanthropic organizations and academic institutions must step in. This is not fringe science. It is central to recovery.

We also need coordination. Right now, many teams are running similar studies in isolation. We need shared platforms: Open data, Common symptom measures, Research networks, Multisite collaborations. The WHO, GBD collaborators, and international neurological societies can help lead this effort.

PCNS must also be included in burden of disease estimates: DALY and YLD calculations, Disability metrics, Health impact models. These numbers drive funding, policy, and services. If PCNS is left out, it will be left behind again.

6.25 Moving from Discovery to Impact

Research must not end in journals. It must lead to change. That means translating findings into clinical guidelines, teaching new knowledge to clinicians, updating care pathways, and funding effective programs. Research should also be shared with patients, in plain language, with honesty, and with hope.

We must build registries that track outcomes, dashboards that show progress, and rapid feedback systems that help providers and patients adjust care. Innovation should be connected to action.

The days of research for research's sake are over. Now, we must research to serve.

6.26 The Role of the IGAP Framework

The WHO Intersectoral Global Action Plan gives us a clear model [14–21]. It calls for integration of research, care, education, and data systems. It promotes equity. It encourages governments to invest in neurological health. PCNS fits squarely into this vision.

By aligning our PCNS research priorities with IGAP, we ensure global relevance. We ensure we are not duplicating effort, and we build momentum toward lasting neurological system reform.

The IGAP framework also reminds us to work across sectors. PCNS research should connect with mental health: Public health, Social policy, Education, Disability support. Only then can we fully understand the scale of the issue and develop whole-person responses.

We are not starting from zero. We have tools, teams, early data, and lived experience. What we need now is focus, urgency, leadership, and funding. PCNS research is not just a scientific opportunity. It is a moral obligation.

People are waiting, not just for answers, but for hope. Let us not delay. Let us research with purpose, with partnership, with precision.

And let us make sure that when answers come, they reach those who need them most.

6.27 Discussion

The emergence of Post COVID-19 Neurological Syndrome has revealed a gap in how we approach, define, and respond to complex neurological conditions that follow systemic infections. Despite the strong patient voices, rising clinical reports, and increasing research interest, PCNS remains largely unrecognized in most health systems. This delay in acknowledgment has had consequences. People are suffering without access to coordinated care, clear explanations, or meaningful treatment plans.

What we have learned from patients in Australia, the UK, the USA, and beyond is consistent. The symptoms are persistent, disabling, and often invisible to standard investigations. Patients are being dismissed or told to "wait it out." They are seeing specialists who may not fully understand the condition. They are referred from one service to another without a clear pathway. Most importantly, they are doing this while struggling with memory loss, brain fog, pain, and exhaustion. This is not just inefficient. It is harmful.

The problem is not simply that PCNS is difficult to treat. The problem is that we have not defined it properly. We have not invested in services to meet the need. We have not trained clinicians to recognize it. We have not yet built the research structures to explore the biology behind it. What we are doing is not enough, and patients know it.

This chapter has proposed a new direction. One grounded in three pillars: services, education, and research. These are not abstract ideas. They are concrete actions. We need clinics that bring multiple disciplines together to support recovery. We need education for every level of the healthcare system and beyond. We need to fund research that asks the right questions and measures what truly matters to patients.

Walking with patients and families must be our starting point. PCNS is not just a post-viral complication. It is a lived neurological syndrome that affects the whole person. Our response must match that complexity with compassion and coordination.

6.28 Conclusion

Post COVID-19 Neurological Syndrome is not a mystery. It is a global neurological crisis that demands structured, science-based, and patient-informed action. The suffering is real. The burden is measurable. The science is emerging, but the systems to address it remain underdeveloped and disconnected.

This chapter has argued for three pillars (services, education, and research) as the foundation of an effective response to PCNS, but these pillars cannot be built in isolation. We urgently need collaboration across disciplines and institutions. Multiple universities must work together. Basic science laboratories, public health researchers, and clinical scientists need to share knowledge, align data, and pursue meaningful questions about causation, progression, and treatment.

Equally, this effort cannot be limited to academic centers. Frontline clinicians in both primary and tertiary care must be at the table. They see these patients daily. Their insights are critical for building practical, scalable, and equitable care models. Patients and carers must not be consulted after the fact, they must be engaged from the beginning as true partners in co-design, governance, and evaluation.

This is the only way to generate trust, build real-world solutions, and translate discovery into relief. PCNS is a whole-person condition. Our response must reflect that. Cross-sector, patient-centered, and globally aligned collaboration is not optional it is essential.

Let us name it, study it, support it, and build what people need, together.

References

1. Wijeratne T, Crewther S. Post-COVID 19 Neurological Syndrome (PCNS); a novel syndrome with challenges for the global neurology community. J Neurol Sci. 2020;419:117179.
2. Turk F, Sweetman J, Chew-Graham CA, Gabbay M, Shepherd J, van der Feltz-Cornelis C, et al. Accessing care for long Covid from the perspectives of patients and healthcare practitioners: a qualitative study. Health Expect. 2024;27:e14008.
3. Dani M, Dirksen A, Taraborrelli P, Torocastro M, Panagopoulos D, Sutton R, Lim PB. Autonomic dysfunction in 'long COVID': rationale, physiology and management strategies. Clin Med. 2021;21:e63–7.
4. Peiris S, Izcovich A, Ordunez P, Luciani S, Martinez C, Aldighieri S, Reveiz L. Challenges to delivering evidence-based management for long COVID. BMJ Evid Based Med. 2023;28:295–8.
5. Voruz P, Assal F, Peron JA. The economic burden of the post-COVID-19 condition: underestimated long-term consequences of neuropsychological deficits. J Glob Health. 2023;13:03019.
6. Heneka MT, Golenbock D, Latz E, Morgan D, Brown R. Immediate and long-term consequences of COVID-19 infections for the development of neurological disease. Alzheimer's Res Ther. 2020;12:69.
7. Kwon J, Milne R, Rayner C, Rocha Lawrence R, Mullard J, Mir G, et al. Impact of long COVID on productivity and informal caregiving. Eur J Health Econ. 2024;25:1095–115.
8. Kim Y, Bae S, Chang HH, Kim SW. Long COVID prevalence and impact on quality of life 2 years after acute COVID-19. Sci Rep. 2023;13:11207.
9. Xu E, Xie Y, Al-Aly Z. Long-term neurologic outcomes of COVID-19. Nat Med. 2022;28:2406–15.

10. Molnar T, Lehoczki A, Fekete M, Varnai R, Zavori L, Erdo-Bonyar S, et al. Mitochondrial dysfunction in long COVID: mechanisms, consequences, and potential therapeutic approaches. GeroScience. 2024;46:5267–86.
11. Woodrow M, Carey C, Ziauddeen N, Thomas R, Akrami A, Lutje V, et al. Systematic review of the prevalence of long COVID. Open Forum Infect Dis. 2023;10
12. Gross M, Lansang NM, Gopaul U, Ogawa EF, Heyn PC, Santos FH, et al. What do I need to know about long-Covid-related fatigue, brain fog, and mental health changes? Arch Phys Med Rehabil. 2023;104:996–1002.
13. Schmachtenberg T, Königs G, Dragaqina A, Roder S, Müller F, Müllenmeister C, et al. Experiences of people with long COVID regarding medical care and barriers in the German healthcare system. BMC Health Serv Res. 2023;23:1160.
14. Pai AA, Young-Sing Q, Bera S, Maheshwari K, Misra A. Analysis of clinical and patient-reported outcomes in post-ELAPE perineal reconstruction with IGAP flap. JPRAS Open. 2022;34:10–20.
15. Leitinger M, Klampfer C, Obermeyr L, Orav K, Damavandi PT, Alexa M, et al. Epilepsy and employment: a qualitative interview study with heads of human resources and occupational physicians in Austria. Epilepsia. 2025;66:712–24.
16. Sen A, Newton CR, Ngwende G. Epilepsy in low- to middle-income countries. Curr Opin Neurol. 2025;38:121–7.
17. Grisold W, Freedman M, Gouider R, Guekht A, Lewis S, Medina M, et al. The Intersectoral Global Action Plan (IGAP): a unique opportunity for neurology across the globe. J Neurol Sci. 2023;449:120645.
18. Reynolds EH. The origins and early development of the ILAE/IBE/WHO global campaign against epilepsy: out of the shadows. Epilepsia Open. 2024;9:77–83.
19. Bharti SK, Gupta I, Akshima, Madaan P, Devi N, Dhir P, et al. Societal costs of illness for infantile epileptic spasms syndrome and evolutionary cost prediction in the era of WHO's IGAP. Epilepsy Res. 2024;199:107284.
20. Wijeratne T, Sales C, Wijeratne C, Karimi L, Jakovljevic M. Systematic review of existing stroke guidelines: case for a change. Biomed Res Int. 2022;2022:5514793.
21. Wasay M, Younis S, Charway-Felli A, Basri H. WHO's Intersectoral Global Action Plan (IGAP); implications for Asian and African countries. J Neurol Sci. 2023;444:120499.

7 Education in Post-COVID Neurological Syndrome (PCNS)

Vimukthi Pathiraja, Tissa Wijeratne,
and Reuben Parama Iswara

7.1 Introduction: Why Education Is Central to the Future of PCNS Care

The COVID-19 pandemic has left a lasting mark on every health system in the world. While the acute crisis has passed for many, the long-term consequences continue to unfold. One of the most significant of these is Post COVID-19 Neurological Syndrome, or PCNS. This condition has emerged as a serious and disabling aftermath for many individuals who had COVID-19, regardless of the severity of their initial infection. It is now clear that PCNS is not rare. It is common. It is debilitating, and most importantly, it is not being managed well.

A major reason for this gap is a lack of education. In every setting, from primary care to tertiary hospitals, clinicians report confusion and uncertainty when faced with PCNS. Patients are presenting with memory issues, fatigue, headaches, dizziness, and emotional instability, yet many clinicians have not received any formal training on how to identify or manage these symptoms in the context of a post-viral neurological condition. This has led to widespread misdiagnosis, inconsistent care, and patient distress.

This chapter begins with a simple idea. If we want to improve outcomes for people living with PCNS, we must first educate those responsible for their care. Education is not an optional extra. It is the foundation on which every other part of

V. Pathiraja (✉)
North Coburg Medical Centre, Coburg North, VIC, Australia

T. Wijeratne
Department of Neurology and Stroke, La Trobe University, St. Albans, VIC, Australia
e-mail: tissa.wijeratne@wh.org.au

R. Parama Iswara
Department of Neurology, Western Health, Melbourne, VIC, Australia
e-mail: Reuben.ParamaIswara@wh.org.au

T. Wijeratne, S. Crewther (eds.), *Post Covid-19 Neurological Syndrome*,
https://doi.org/10.1007/978-3-032-14995-4_7

the response must be built. Without knowledge, there is no diagnosis. Without training, there is no coordinated care. Without understanding, there is no empathy.

The need for targeted education spans all levels of the healthcare system. Medical students are not being taught about PCNS in their foundational training. General practitioners are trying to support patients without diagnostic tools or referral pathways. Specialists are often seeing patients late in their illness, after many months of unmanaged symptoms. Allied health professionals—physiotherapists, psychologists, occupational therapists—are being called upon to support rehabilitation but have limited knowledge of the underlying pathophysiology or pacing principles unique to PCNS.

This is a failure of the system, not of individuals. We cannot expect clinicians to treat what they have never been taught to recognize. We cannot ask them to guide recovery if they do not understand the condition, and we cannot achieve consistency in care until we create a shared base of knowledge.

The need is not the same everywhere. In high-income countries, there are often advanced medical education systems, but content on PCNS is still lacking. In low-income and resource-limited settings, the challenge is more complex. There may be fewer neurologists, limited access to diagnostic testing, and even greater reliance on community health workers and generalists, yet the burden of PCNS in these settings is no less real. If anything, the social and economic consequences of untreated PCNS may be greater where safety nets are weaker and access to care more limited.

That is why PCNS education must be context-specific. In some settings, the focus will be on specialist training and continuing professional development. In others, the priority will be basic awareness and syndromic recognition in the absence of testing. In all cases, the aim must be to equip health workers with practical, compassionate, and actionable skills. They must be able to recognize red flags. Know when to refer and understand how to support recovery over time.

But education must go beyond the clinical workforce. Public health professionals, educators, social workers, and disability support teams also need a working knowledge of PCNS. They must understand how it affects school attendance, employment, family dynamics, and mental health. Without this broader awareness, patients continue to face disbelief, stigma, and isolation.

Universities and teaching hospitals have a critical role to play. They must rapidly update their curricula to reflect emerging evidence on PCNS. Clinical rotations should include exposure to post-viral and neurological rehabilitation. Final-year projects and dissertations should focus on real-world PCNS challenges. Academic journals must encourage the publication of teaching case series and best practice models. This cannot be left to informal learning or patient-led advocacy alone.

Most importantly, we must bring together multiple sectors to build a responsive and resilient education platform. This includes universities, health departments, professional colleges, and accreditation bodies. Basic science researchers must work closely with public health educators. Primary care clinicians must be part of the discussion with specialists, and patients must help design the educational content itself. They are the best teachers of what PCNS feels like, what it disrupts, and what helps.

Education must also be ongoing. PCNS is a new condition, and our understanding is still evolving. What we teach today may need to be updated tomorrow. That is why all training must include mechanisms for revision, feedback, and reflection. We must build learning systems that grow with the science and remain rooted in the real experiences of patients and carers.

In the chapters that follow, we will explore the core competencies needed for PCNS care. We will outline practical steps to integrate PCNS into existing training programs. We will present case studies from different parts of the world, and we will make the case that education is not just a support strategy, it is a central pillar in addressing one of the most urgent neurological syndromes of our time.

The opportunity is here. The challenge is clear. The time to act is now.

7.2 Understanding the Educational Imperative for PCNS

Post COVID-19 Neurological Syndrome is now recognized as a serious and disabling condition. It affects millions of people across the world. Unlike typical post-viral recovery, PCNS is complex and unpredictable. Symptoms can persist for months or even years. They include brain fog, memory loss, fatigue, sleep problems, headaches, emotional changes, and nervous system instability. These symptoms may come and go. They may change over time. And they often overlap. This creates a confusing and frustrating experience for patients and clinicians alike.

To address this, we must focus on education. Doctors, nurses, physiotherapists, psychologists, and other health professionals need better training. Without it, PCNS will continue to be misdiagnosed, misunderstood, and mismanaged. Health professionals must be equipped to identify symptoms early. They must also understand how to support patients over time. This requires both clinical knowledge and compassionate communication.

PCNS does not present in a predictable pattern. A person may appear well but feel unwell. Their scans may be normal, but they may struggle to think clearly, sleep, or manage their daily routine. Because of this, standard tools may not detect the problem. Education must teach clinicians how to listen carefully. They must be trained to validate symptoms, not dismiss them. Early recognition leads to better outcomes.

Training must also reflect the wide range of symptoms. Cognitive impairment, for example, is not just about memory loss. It includes difficulty concentrating, reduced mental stamina, word-finding problems, and trouble with multitasking. Fatigue in PCNS is not ordinary tiredness. It is a deep physical and mental exhaustion. It can be triggered by minor exertion and may take days to recover from. This is not laziness or depression. It is a neurological issue.

Headaches in PCNS are also unique. Some resemble migraines. Others feel like a constant pressure. Some patients describe burning or tingling pain in the head or face. Health workers must learn to differentiate these from more common headache types. They must also understand that typical treatments may not work.

Sleep issues in PCNS are another major concern. Many patients cannot fall asleep easily. Others wake frequently during the night. Some sleep for long hours but still feel unrefreshed. Traditional sleep aids may not help. Sleep problems also worsen other symptoms. When a patient with PCNS does not sleep, their brain fog, pain, and mood symptoms usually intensify.

Autonomic dysfunction is another key feature. This means the body's automatic systems—like heart rate, blood pressure, and digestion—are out of balance. Patients may feel dizzy when standing up. They may experience rapid heartbeat after eating. They may feel hot or cold at odd times. These symptoms are often overlooked or mistaken for anxiety. Education can help clinicians understand these signs and avoid unnecessary referrals or mislabeling.

Mental health symptoms are often the most misunderstood. PCNS patients may feel anxious, tearful, or emotionally flat. Some experience sudden mood swings or panic attacks, but these symptoms are not always psychological in origin. They may be driven by changes in brain chemistry or inflammation. Treating them requires a combined neurological and psychological approach.

Training must also address communication skills. Many patients have been dismissed or doubted. They are told it is "just stress" or "post-viral fatigue." This kind of dismissal leads to isolation and hopelessness. Clinicians must learn how to build trust. They must take time to explain what is known—and what is not yet known. They must partner with the patient in decision-making.

Another essential area is pacing. Many people with PCNS get worse after activity. This is called post-exertional symptom exacerbation. It happens after too much walking, talking, or even thinking. Patients may feel fine during the activity but crash hours or days later. Clinicians must be trained in how to help patients balance activity and rest. This includes using pacing tools, helping set limits, and recognizing signs of overexertion.

Care also needs to be adapted across income settings. In low-resource settings, health professionals may not have access to advanced testing or specialised clinics. Training in these areas must focus on clinical signs, history taking, and syndromic diagnosis. Community health workers and nurses should be trained to identify common PCNS symptoms and provide support at the local level.

In high-resource settings, more tools may be available. Yet even here, education is lacking. Many specialists do not yet consider PCNS a neurological issue. They may treat individual symptoms but miss the larger pattern. Multidisciplinary training can help bridge these gaps. It encourages collaboration across neurology, rehabilitation, psychiatry, general practice, and allied health.

Medical schools and training institutions have a role to play. PCNS should be included in undergraduate and postgraduate teaching. Continuing professional development should include sessions on post-viral conditions. Short online courses, clinical tip sheets, and case-based learning modules should be developed and shared widely.

Universities must also promote collaboration between basic scientists and clinicians. Research on neuroinflammation, immune pathways, and autonomic dysfunction must be linked to clinical observations. When scientists and frontline workers talk to each other, they can build better models of care. They can also help translate new discoveries into real-world solutions.

Public health educators must be involved as well. PCNS has implications beyond the clinic. It affects employment, education, disability services, and public awareness. Public health training should include content on the social and economic impact of PCNS and how to respond with inclusive policies.

Finally, patients and carers must be involved in education. They bring insights that no textbook can teach. They know how the illness feels. What makes it better. What makes it worse. Their voice should shape curriculum design, training sessions, and clinical simulations.

Education for PCNS is not about adding more content. It is about changing the culture. It is about shifting from scepticism to understanding. From passive treatment to active listening. From isolated care to coordinated support. The more we teach this, the more lives we can help rebuild.

7.3 Early Detection and Diagnosis

Timely diagnosis is one of the most important steps in managing Post COVID-19 Neurological Syndrome. Early recognition can help prevent unnecessary suffering. It can also improve the chances of recovery and reduce long-term disability.

Unfortunately, many patients with PCNS are not diagnosed early. Some are not diagnosed at all. They go from one doctor to another. They hear different opinions. They are told to rest, reduce stress, or exercise. Many are told their symptoms are psychological. This leads to delayed care and deep frustration.

We must change this. The first step is education. Healthcare professionals need to know what to look for. They need clear guidance on how to recognize the early signs of PCNS, and they must understand that early detection is not just helpful. It is essential.

7.4 Recognizing Early Symptoms

PCNS can begin with subtle symptoms. A person may report feeling off. They might struggle with memory. They may feel more tired than usual. They might complain of headaches, dizziness, or a heavy feeling in the head. Some describe sensory overload. Others say they just don't feel like themselves.

These signs can be missed if clinicians are not trained to connect the dots. That is why education must include practical symptom recognition. Every general practitioner, emergency doctor, nurse, and allied health worker must learn how PCNS typically presents, not just in textbooks, but in real patients.

This training must also reach primary care clinics. In most places, that is where patients first seek help. General practitioners play a critical role, but many do not yet feel confident identifying PCNS. We need simple checklists, clinical guides, and decision tools to help them.

Training must also reach emergency departments and hospital outpatient clinics. These are high-pressure environments. Symptoms like brain fog or dizziness may be dismissed as minor, but for the patient, they are life-altering. Awareness among triage staff and junior doctors is crucial, especially because patients often feel embarrassed to bring up what they are experiencing.

We also need to include public health networks. Primary Health Networks in Australia, for example, can help distribute training materials and create referral pathways. Health authorities can also support awareness campaigns so that clinicians do not feel they are working in isolation.

7.5 Diagnostic Tools and Clinical Evaluation

Once symptoms are recognized, the next step is evaluation. There is no single test for PCNS. Diagnosis is based on history, symptom patterns, exclusion of other conditions, and functional assessment. Clinicians must be trained in how to do this carefully.

History taking must include questions about previous COVID-19 infection. The severity of the initial illness does not predict PCNS risk. Even mild or asymptomatic infections can lead to long-term neurological symptoms. This must be part of the diagnostic thinking.

We also need structured tools. Screening forms can help document symptoms like brain fog, fatigue, orthostatic intolerance, or emotional changes. These forms should be easy to use. They should work in different settings, from general practice to neurology clinics.

Cognitive screening tools can be helpful, but they must be used wisely. Many PCNS patients have normal scores on standard tests, yet they still struggle with everyday tasks. Clinicians need to know that a normal test does not rule out PCNS. Functional assessment is just as important. Can the patient work? Drive? Read a book? Hold a conversation in a noisy room?

Testing for autonomic dysfunction is another key area. Many PCNS patients develop POTS or other forms of dysautonomia. Training should include how to do a basic active stand test. This can be done in any clinic. It provides vital clues about the patient's nervous system stability.

In some cases, further testing may be needed. Brain imaging, blood tests, and ECGs can help rule out other causes, but clinicians must be taught that normal results do not mean nothing is wrong. PCNS is a syndrome of functional disruption. It may not show up on standard scans.

We must also develop new tools. Digital health solutions could support early detection. For example, a mobile app could help patients track symptoms and know when to seek care. These tools could also help clinicians by summarizing patterns or flagging red flags.

Artificial intelligence may also help in the future, but for now, the most powerful tool remains clinical judgment, and clinical judgment improves with training, exposure, and listening to patients.

7.6 Bringing Early Detection into the Real World

We must move beyond theory. Early diagnosis must happen in the real world. That means adapting training for different levels of the system.

In rural areas, nurses and community health workers should be trained to spot PCNS symptoms. In urban settings, hospital triage protocols should include basic PCNS screening questions. In allied health, physiotherapists and psychologists should know how to recognize patterns that suggest deeper neurological dysfunction.

Education must also include when to refer. General practitioners must know where to send patients for further evaluation. Health systems must create referral hubs or centres of excellence for PCNS. Without this, patients will continue to fall between services.

Public health bodies must also support this work. Information campaigns can help patients understand their symptoms. Early self-recognition can lead to earlier help-seeking. This reduces delay and distress.

Digital health platforms can also support shared learning. Online modules, webinars, and case libraries can be accessed by health professionals in any setting. They can update their knowledge in their own time. This helps scale the training effort quickly.

7.7 Involving Patients in Diagnostic Education

Patients must be part of this process. They know what it feels like to be dismissed. Their insights can help shape diagnostic training. Case studies, simulations, videos, all can include real patient voices.

Patients can also help identify what symptoms are most disabling and most often overlooked. This can shape how we teach symptom clusters and case recognition. Education must reflect lived reality, not just clinical language.

Finally, we must measure progress. Health systems should track how many clinicians are trained. How many PCNS cases are being identified. How long it takes from first symptoms to diagnosis. These data can help improve the system.

7.8 Comprehensive Patient Management

Education in PCNS must cover various aspects of patient care, from clinical assessment to rehabilitation and follow-up. Healthcare professionals should be knowledgeable about:

- *Multidisciplinary care approaches*: Understanding how to collaborate with neurologists, psychologists, physical therapists, and other specialists to provide holistic care.

- *Treatment and management strategies*: Training on both pharmacological and non-pharmacological approaches for managing PCNS symptoms.

7.9 Educational Needs for Healthcare Professionals

The burden of Post COVID-19 Neurological Syndrome (PCNS) is growing, yet many healthcare workers still lack the knowledge to diagnose and manage it. This gap affects both high-income and low-income countries. Clinicians in both settings face challenges. Some have too many resources to choose from. Others have almost none. What they share is the need for clarity and structure.

Training is key. We must help clinicians to spot PCNS symptoms early. They must know how to ask the right questions. They must know what to look for during an exam, and they must know when to refer a patient for more help. Without these skills, patients may be misdiagnosed. They may receive inappropriate care, or worse, they may be told their symptoms are not real.

There are core skills that every clinician must have. First, they must be able to take a clear history of neurological symptoms. They must ask about fatigue, brain fog, dizziness, memory problems, and sensory issues. Next, they must do a focused neurological exam. This should include basic motor, sensory, cranial nerve, and coordination checks. Clinicians must also learn how to assess cognitive function in a simple and quick way.

Communication is another core skill. Patients with PCNS often feel dismissed. Clinicians must listen carefully. They must explain the diagnosis clearly. They must involve patients in decisions. A trusting relationship improves outcomes.

One proposed solution is to develop standard PCNS training modules. These can be used in medical schools. They can also be part of ongoing professional development. These modules should be simple, evidence-based, and practical. They must also be updated as new knowledge emerges.

Simulation-based training can also help. Using case studies and virtual scenarios improves learning. Clinicians can practice identifying PCNS. They can test out treatment plans. They can improve how they talk to patients.

Education must be matched to local resources. In low-income settings, simple decision-making tools are useful. In high-resource settings, digital diagnostic tools and biomarkers may be added. The Royal Australian College of Physicians and similar bodies can play a role. They can help set standards and provide accreditation. General practice colleges can also support training in primary care settings.

Many clinicians in LMICs may never have heard of PCNS. This is not their fault. It is the result of poor dissemination of global knowledge. There must be more outreach. We need regional training hubs, online open-access courses, workshops at conferences, and support from global neurology organizations.

The WHO Intersectoral Global Action Plan on epilepsy and other neurological disorders (IGAP) calls for stronger neurology training worldwide [2, 11]. PCNS fits this mandate. It is a neurological disorder that affects millions. It requires the same investment as stroke, epilepsy, and dementia. A recent white paper from the World Federation of Neurology also highlights this gap [1].

Finally, education must include a focus on equity. Many patients are women. Many come from racial or ethnic minorities. Many have mental health needs. Training must include trauma-informed care, cultural humility, and an understanding of social determinants of health. Only then can we meet the true needs of our patients.

7.10 Educational Requirements in Low-Income Settings

Low-income countries face unique challenges in delivering healthcare. These challenges are even more significant when it comes to training clinicians in new and complex conditions such as Post COVID-19 Neurological Syndrome (PCNS). A lack of infrastructure, trained specialists, and educational materials can delay or prevent diagnosis and care, yet the need is urgent. Millions of people in low-resource settings are experiencing the long-term effects of COVID-19 without support or recognition.

One of the biggest barriers is the lack of specialist neurology services. In many countries, there may be only a handful of neurologists for millions of people. Therefore, the responsibility of recognizing PCNS often falls to general practitioners, nurses, and community health workers. These primary care providers need targeted training that fits their context and workload.

Basic neurological training must be the foundation. Clinicians must learn to take a good history. They must be taught to ask about fatigue, memory loss, dizziness, and headaches. They must know that these symptoms may represent PCNS and not just stress or weakness. Training should include simple neurological assessments that can be done without special tools.

Clear referral protocols are also essential. Primary care workers must be trained to recognize when to refer a patient to higher levels of care. This is especially true for cases with red flags such as severe headache, visual changes, weakness, or confusion. Structured pathways help avoid delays in care.

One solution is to integrate PCNS training into existing primary care education. Ministries of health, medical schools, and NGOs can collaborate to create modules. These can be delivered in person or online. Local language versions will help improve understanding. Case-based learning using real patient stories can make the material more relatable and effective.

Peer education models can also be helpful. Experienced primary care workers can be trained as “PCNS champions.” They can then train others in their clinics or regions. This approach has been used successfully in other global health programs, including epilepsy and mental health.

Access to continuing professional development is another priority. For example, mobile apps can be used to deliver educational updates. Text message reminders and simple guides can reinforce learning. Radio programs or short educational videos can reach rural providers.

The World Health Organization (WHO) encourages integrated training programs as part of its Intersectoral Global Action Plan on neurological disorders [2, 11]. This plan emphasizes task-sharing, capacity-building, and access to neurological care at all levels. It also recommends community engagement and local leadership to adapt global knowledge to national contexts.

Collaborative models such as Project ECHO (Extension for Community Healthcare Outcomes) may offer value. In this model, a central team of specialists provides regular video-based mentoring to primary care providers in remote settings. This has been used for a variety of diseases and may suit PCNS education.

Educational materials must also be culturally appropriate. In some countries, symptoms like fatigue or brain fog may be misunderstood. Local beliefs about illness must be respected and addressed with care. A strong link between science and community trust must be built.

In summary, low-income settings require low-cost, high-impact education strategies to manage PCNS. These strategies must focus on frontline health workers. They must be practical, scalable, and locally adapted. Without investment in training, early detection and care will remain out of reach for millions. This is both a scientific and moral challenge.

7.11 Utilizing Community Health Workers

Community health workers (CHWs) are vital in low-income countries. They often serve as the first and only point of contact for healthcare. In managing Post COVID-19 Neurological Syndrome (PCNS), CHWs can play a big role. They can help with early recognition, patient support, and education.

Training CHWs is practical and effective. Short workshops can teach them to identify key PCNS symptoms. These include fatigue, brain fog, mood changes, and ongoing headaches. Teaching should focus on observation and communication. Many CHWs already know their communities well. With proper tools, they can link patients to higher levels of care.

Hands-on training should be prioritized. Simple exercises in villages or community centres can improve confidence and skill. Trainers can use posters, flipbooks, or videos in local languages.

Mobile training units can reach remote areas. These are vans or teams that travel with materials and trainers. They are already used for programs in maternal health, tuberculosis, and vaccination. They should now include neurological health and PCNS awareness.

Smartphone apps can help too. Many CHWs have mobile phones. Apps can show common symptoms and how to separate PCNS from infections like malaria or tuberculosis. Simple decision trees or quizzes can support learning on the go.

By including CHWs in PCNS care, healthcare systems can extend their reach. This creates trust, improves early detection, and supports families close to home.

7.12 Distance Learning and Technology-Based Solutions

In many low-resource settings, specialists are rare. Travel is costly and time-consuming. This is why distance learning and digital tools are key to training more health workers.

E-learning platforms are a cost-effective solution. Free or low-cost courses can help doctors, nurses, and CHWs. These platforms must be mobile-friendly and available offline. They should offer short modules on PCNS basics, red flags, and management tips. Content in local languages is essential.

Tele-mentoring is another powerful tool. Programs like Project ECHO show how local providers can learn from experts without leaving their communities. In these programs, groups of providers meet online to discuss real cases. They get advice from neurologists, psychiatrists, or rehabilitation experts. Over time, their skills improve, and patients receive better care.

Interactive learning is more effective than lectures alone. Video-based simulations, case studies, and quizzes can make education more practical. Platforms like WhatsApp or Telegram can support peer-to-peer learning and rapid communication.

Governments, NGOs, and universities should invest in these tools. Partnerships with international health agencies can help develop high-quality PCNS training for low-income settings.

By combining local talent with global support, technology can reduce the education gap. It can make PCNS care better, even where doctors and clinics are few.

7.13 Educational Requirements in High-Income Settings

In high-income countries, healthcare systems have more capacity. There are better diagnostic tools, more specialists, and advanced clinical training programs. However, PCNS remains under-recognized. This makes education about PCNS just as essential in these settings as anywhere else.

7.14 Advanced Training Programs

Advanced clinical education should now include dedicated content on PCNS. At present, few formal curricula cover post-viral neurological syndromes in detail. This is a missed opportunity. Structured fellowships in neuroimmunology, neurorehabilitation, and long COVID care should be expanded. Certification programs can also support primary care and allied health professionals.

Interdisciplinary workshops are important. They can bring together neurologists, rehabilitation physicians, general practitioners, psychologists, and nurses. Sharing experience improves coordinated care. For example, headache specialists and autonomic clinics can contribute valuable expertise.

Hospitals should also support case-based teaching. Case rounds that focus on PCNS can deepen clinical understanding. Simulation-based training should be explored as a tool to teach symptom management, communication, and shared decision-making.

Medical colleges like the Royal Australasian College of Physicians and Royal College of General Practitioners should incorporate PCNS into ongoing professional development. Including PCNS content in continuing medical education will support broader system awareness.

7.15 Research and Evidence-Based Practice

High-income countries must lead in building the evidence base for PCNS care. This requires training clinicians not just as care providers, but as contributors to research.

Educational institutions should offer training in research methods that are relevant to PCNS. These can include cohort study design, biomarker analysis, neuroimaging interpretation, and patient-reported outcome measures. Clinicians must also learn how to critically appraise emerging studies on PCNS interventions.

Access to updated information is crucial. Libraries, medical societies, and universities must ensure clinicians can access journals, webinars, and conferences. Subscription-based journals should provide open access to PCNS content when possible. Educational campaigns can also help combat misinformation about PCNS, which has been common throughout the pandemic.

High-income countries should also facilitate clinician involvement in multicentre trials. This includes trials on medications, cognitive rehabilitation, mental health interventions, and autonomic therapies. Research training should highlight ethical recruitment, patient partnership, and equity in trial design.

Academic centers should partner with patient advocacy groups. This ensures that research addresses patient priorities. It also supports culturally responsive and trauma-informed care.

Lastly, mentorship programs should be created to guide young clinicians interested in PCNS. These can help grow the next generation of experts in neuro-COVID care.

Collaboration between high-income and low-income countries offers a powerful opportunity for mutual growth. While high-income nations possess advanced research infrastructure and clinical trial capacity, they often lack exposure to the broader diversity of disease expression seen in lower-resource settings. Partnering with low-income countries allows for a richer understanding of PCNS presentations, especially in communities with high exposure to environmental stressors and limited access to early COVID-19 care. Such collaborations also promote resource-conscious clinical decision-making. By learning to choose wisely and implement scalable, cost-effective models, high-income countries can develop more sustainable and equitable approaches to care. Conversely, low-income countries benefit from access to diagnostics, training, and scientific exchange. Together, these partnerships foster a win-win model—advancing both global brain health equity and scientific innovation. As emphasized in the WHO IGAP and Brain Health Position Paper, shared learning and solidarity are essential to bridging the neurological divide [2, 11]. It is through cooperation, not competition, that we will collectively address the burden of PCNS and strengthen global resilience against future neurological health crises.

7.16 Interdisciplinary Collaboration in PCNS Education

Post COVID-19 Neurological Syndrome (PCNS) is a complex disorder. It affects the brain, the immune system, and many body functions. Managing PCNS requires input from many healthcare professionals. Neurologists, rehabilitation experts, psychologists, general practitioners, and allied health workers must all be involved. Each brings a different skill set. Together, they can deliver better care, but this only works if they understand each other's roles. That is why interdisciplinary education is vital.

Interdisciplinary education trains teams to think and act together. It encourages respect across professions. It teaches collaboration from the start. This approach must be embedded in undergraduate, postgraduate, and continuing education.

Team-based learning is one model. In this approach, students or professionals from different fields work together on the same case. They learn to plan care as a group. Case studies can reflect real-life PCNS scenarios. For example, a patient with brain fog, fatigue, and anxiety may need input from a neurologist, a psychologist, and a physiotherapist. Working together, the team develops a care plan that covers all aspects of the illness.

Inter-professional education (IPE) is another proven strategy. It teaches students from different fields in the same classroom or clinical setting. Medical, nursing, and allied health students learn side by side. They learn how each discipline thinks. They also learn when to refer and when to lead. Research shows IPE improves communication and reduces errors [7]. It also makes teams more efficient and empathetic.

Training should also focus on common tools and language. For example, standard outcome measures for fatigue or cognitive function should be known to all team members. This ensures everyone is talking about the same issues and using the same metrics.

Leadership training is important too. PCNS care often lacks a single lead clinician. Team leaders need skills to coordinate care and maintain trust. Regular team meetings, shared care records, and open communication are essential. These are skills that can be taught and practiced.

Digital tools can help. Shared electronic records allow all providers to view the patient's progress. Apps and platforms can host care plans, schedules, and updates, but technology alone is not enough. Teams must also build relationships and trust.

Ongoing professional development should include interdisciplinary workshops. These can cover new research, guidelines, or treatments. They also offer a space for peer learning and sharing of best practices.

Finally, patients and families should be part of the team. Education must train professionals to include them in decision-making. PCNS care is long-term and often unpredictable. Empowering patients with knowledge and tools improves outcomes.

In summary, interdisciplinary collaboration is not optional in PCNS care. It is a core requirement. Education systems must invest in training that builds these skills early and often. Only then can teams deliver the integrated care that PCNS patients need.

7.17 Communication Skills Development in PCNS Education

Effective communication is central to quality care in Post COVID-19 Neurological Syndrome (PCNS). It shapes how teams work together. It also shapes how patients understand and manage their illness. In PCNS, where symptoms are diverse and long-lasting, communication must be clear, compassionate, and consistent.

Many patients with PCNS feel dismissed. They describe being misunderstood or told their symptoms are psychological. Others report that their care is fragmented. This is often due to poor communication between healthcare providers. It leads to duplicated tests, missed referrals, and frustration for both patients and clinicians. Better communication can fix this. It is not a soft skill. It is a core clinical competency.

Healthcare professionals must be trained to communicate across roles. Neurologists must explain symptoms to psychologists. Nurses must report concerns to rehabilitation teams. Occupational therapists must understand physician care plans. This is only possible when professionals speak the same language. Training must promote shared understanding.

One approach is case conferencing. Case conferences bring professionals together. Each shares their observations. Each learns from others. This builds a team mindset. It also ensures that patient care is coherent. Practice with case conferencing should be included in all training programs. Students and trainees should learn how to present, listen, and collaborate.

Role-play is another useful tool. It allows learners to rehearse difficult conversations. For example, how to explain chronic symptoms when there is no diagnostic test, or how to tell a patient that a therapy has failed. These moments are common in PCNS care. Training should not ignore them.

Active listening is essential. It means more than hearing words. It means understanding emotions and values. It means asking open questions. It also means giving patients time to speak. Many PCNS patients need to tell long stories. Their symptoms often shift. Their medical records may be complex. A rushed consultation will miss key details. Listening is both diagnostic and therapeutic.

Written communication also matters. Clear clinic letters and referral notes prevent delays. They support continuity of care. They must be accurate and jargon-free. Training must teach how to write effectively. This includes summarising patient concerns, listing symptoms, and explaining plans.

Digital communication is now common. Telehealth, emails, and electronic records are part of daily care. Professionals must be trained to use these tools well. For instance, video calls must allow space for emotional cues. Written messages must be clear and respectful. Patients often judge their care based on how they are spoken to.

Patient-centred communication is the goal. It means involving patients in decisions. It means asking what matters to them. It means checking understanding. This is especially important in PCNS. Many patients are unsure why they are unwell. Others feel guilt, fear, or anger. They may be coping with job loss, stigma, or uncertainty. These feelings must be addressed. Communication must show empathy.

Cultural competence is part of good communication. Patients may come from different backgrounds. They may use different words for illness. They may have beliefs about healing. Clinicians must respect this. They must avoid assumptions. They must explain care plans in culturally relevant ways.

Family members should also be included. In PCNS, especially in children and older adults, families are key partners. They manage appointments. They support daily routines. They may also feel anxious or confused. Communication must include them, but it must also respect the patient's privacy and voice.

Training must continue after graduation. Workshops, feedback, and mentorship help improve skills. Communication audits can also help. Teams can review how messages are given and received. They can learn what worked and what failed.

Feedback from patients is valuable. It shows whether communication was clear and helpful. It highlights blind spots. Patient feedback should be part of staff development.

Supervisors should model good communication. Students and junior staff watch their mentors. If they see respectful, clear, and kind exchanges, they will follow. If they see rushed, dismissive, or unclear talk, they will do the same.

Language barriers must be addressed. Interpreter services must be easy to access. Staff should be trained to work with interpreters. Written materials should be available in multiple languages. This is not just about translation. It is about equity.

Emotionally charged conversations are common in PCNS. Patients may be frustrated. They may not feel believed. Clinicians must be calm and honest. Training in emotional regulation helps. Burnout can affect communication. Staff need support too.

In summary, communication is not an add-on. It is at the heart of good PCNS care. It supports teamwork. It builds trust. It improves outcomes. Education programs must make it a priority. They must include it at all levels of training.

We call for communication skills to be a core standard in all PCNS education frameworks. We urge health systems to reward good communication. We ask researchers to study its impact more. Communication is the glue that holds care together. Without it, no team can function, and no patient can heal.

7.18 Challenges in Implementing PCNS Education

The global effort to improve care for Post COVID-19 Neurological Syndrome (PCNS) faces many challenges. One of the most pressing is the lack of education for healthcare professionals. Teaching healthcare workers about PCNS is essential. Without proper training, patients may be misdiagnosed, dismissed, or poorly managed. The issue is more serious in low-income settings but is relevant across all regions.

Creating good training programs requires money. In many low-income countries, health budgets are already stretched. Education programs, especially new ones, may not get the priority they deserve.

One way to address this is to apply for grants from global health organizations. The World Health Organization (WHO), the Welcome Trust, and non-governmental organizations that focus on public health can help. Governments can also work with private healthcare providers. These public-private partnerships can fund materials, training modules, and digital platforms.

In some cases, private universities or corporate sponsors may be willing to support these initiatives. Local pharmaceutical companies that operate ethically can also help with the distribution of printed materials or support workshops.

In many regions, healthcare providers do not have access to up-to-date materials. Textbooks may be old. Internet access may be limited. Online resources may not be available in local languages.

One solution is to create open-access materials. These can include guides, posters, short video modules, or downloadable content for smartphones. Healthcare workers in remote areas can benefit from audio or video lectures recorded by specialists.

Partnerships with academic institutions can help. Universities in high-income countries can create digital training hubs. These can be accessed by providers across the world, often at no cost. Professional organizations such as the World Federation of Neurology (WFN) can also be involved in content validation and delivery.

Sometimes the problem is not resources but attitude. Healthcare professionals may not want to take part in new training. This can happen when staff are overworked or when they do not yet believe that PCNS is a real condition.

To overcome this, we must make PCNS education easy to access, rewarding, and relevant. Offering continuing medical education (CME) credits is one way to encourage participation. Another approach is to make certification in PCNS management a career-advancing step.

Starting with small pilot programs can help. When doctors and nurses see good results, they are more likely to recommend the program to others. Peer-to-peer learning also works well. Early adopters of PCNS training can become mentors and advocates.

One major barrier is the lack of a standardized PCNS curriculum. What is taught in one country may be different from what is taught in another. This creates confusion and reduces the quality of care.

Creating a global core curriculum could help. Organizations like WHO and WFN could lead this effort. Local health ministries can adapt the curriculum based on resources and need. Topics should include symptoms, differential diagnosis, basic investigations, patient education, and referral pathways.

Case-based learning should also be part of the curriculum. Real-life examples help learners connect theory with practice. These cases should reflect different health system realities, from rural clinics to urban hospitals.

7.19 Language and Cultural Barriers

Many existing materials on PCNS are in English or other widely spoken languages, but healthcare workers often prefer or require training in their native language. Translation and cultural adaptation are crucial.

Materials should be co-developed with local healthcare professionals. They understand which examples and terms will resonate most with their peers. This improves both uptake and understanding.

7.20 Need for Political and Institutional Support

Educational programs cannot succeed without support from health ministries and professional colleges. Advocacy is needed to explain why PCNS matters.

Decision-makers must understand that PCNS is not rare. It affects people of all ages, across all social groups. Its impact on health systems, productivity, and mental health is already significant and growing.

Engaging stakeholders early is key. Ministries of Health, national neurological societies, and public health officials should be invited to contribute to program design and rollout. Their endorsement can make the difference between pilot and scale-up.

7.21 Future Directions: Building Stronger PCNS Education

Looking forward, PCNS education must be flexible, inclusive, and scalable. It must respond to the needs of both healthcare providers and patients. Below are some key recommendations.

Not every professional needs the same depth of training. A modular system lets learners start small and add more as needed. For example, a GP might take a basic PCNS module. Later, they can add advanced sessions on managing dysautonomia or prescribing triptans. This flexibility helps busy professionals engage at their own pace.

Training must include real patient stories. This helps clinicians understand the lived reality of PCNS. Video interviews, anonymized diaries, or patient-led teaching sessions can all be powerful. It also fosters empathy and improves communication.

E-learning platforms are expanding fast. They can host video lectures, quizzes, downloadable handouts, and live webinars. Artificial intelligence may soon offer adaptive learning pathways. For now, even low-tech solutions—like WhatsApp groups for peer support—can be useful in continuing professional development.

Global problems need global solutions. We propose setting up PCNS learning collaboratives that link experts from different regions. These networks can share materials, host joint webinars, and support capacity building. South-South learning is also vital. Countries in the Global South have rich experiences that others can learn from.

PCNS should not be treated as a one-off topic. It should be embedded across disciplines in undergraduate and postgraduate training. For example, medical students should learn about PCNS in neurology, psychiatry, and public health modules. This builds a workforce ready for the future.

7.22 Future Directions and Conclusion

7.22.1 Expanding Digital Learning Platforms

Digital learning offers a powerful way to scale PCNS education. It allows healthcare workers from all regions to access the same high-quality information. This is especially valuable in areas where in-person training is not available.

Online platforms can offer step-by-step learning. They can include clinical videos, voice-over lectures, quizzes, and patient scenarios. These resources should be mobile-friendly and available in multiple languages. Platforms like Moodle or open-source systems can be adapted for local contexts.

Digital tools can also provide on-demand updates. As PCNS knowledge evolves, these updates will keep professionals informed. Public health networks can play a key role in promoting digital education. Ministries of Health, NGOs, and academic institutions should work together to develop and distribute these tools.

7.22.2 Building Collaborative Networks

Collaboration is central to future PCNS education. Working in silos will slow progress. Countries, institutions, and professionals must share knowledge and tools.

International working groups should develop core competencies for PCNS care. These can guide curriculum development globally. They should reflect input from both low-income and high-income settings.

Cross-country exchanges can strengthen understanding. Healthcare workers from high-income countries can learn from innovations in low-resource environments. These often include creative, low-cost solutions. Meanwhile, LMICs benefit from shared access to research and clinical guidelines. This creates a win-win for both sides. It also builds trust and long-term partnerships.

Collaboration should also include patients. Patient organizations can contribute to educational content. They can help ensure materials are clear, relevant, and sensitive to lived experience.

7.22.3 Continuous Evaluation and Improvement

No educational program is perfect from the start. Continuous feedback and evaluation must guide improvement. This includes feedback from frontline healthcare workers and learners themselves.

Simple feedback tools can help. Short surveys, case outcomes, and group discussions provide rich insight. What works in one setting may not work in another. Listening to learners ensures the content stays useful.

Outcomes should be tracked. These can include knowledge gains, improved diagnosis rates, or patient satisfaction. When linked with clinical data, this helps measure real-world impact.

Institutions must commit to regular updates. As the science of PCNS grows, so should the curriculum. Topics like biomarkers, neurorehabilitation, or digital diagnostics may become more central over time. Strong leadership is needed to manage these updates and maintain quality.

7.23 Final Thoughts

PCNS is a global challenge, but it is also an opportunity. It allows us to reimagine how we teach and learn about neurological illness. It pushes us to break silos and work together. The case studies above show what is possible.

In high-income countries, structured certification can raise standards. In low-income settings, community-level interventions can reach those most in need. Technology, creativity, and collaboration are key. So too is a commitment to equity and patient-centered care.

With support from institutions, funders, and communities, we can scale these efforts. By doing so, we not only improve outcomes for PCNS patients—we build a more responsive, inclusive, and resilient health system for the future.

PCNS education is more than a teaching task. It is a global responsibility. Millions of patients are suffering from symptoms that few healthcare workers fully understand. Misinformation and underdiagnosis are common. Education can change this.

To build a workforce ready for PCNS, we need more than books and lectures. We need accessible, flexible, and inclusive training systems. These systems should use digital tools. They should invite collaboration. They should be evaluated regularly.

Digital platforms make education scalable. They can bring expert knowledge to every corner of the world, but tools alone are not enough. Shared learning across countries must be part of the plan. No nation has all the answers. Together, we are stronger.

We must also listen to learners. Healthcare workers face many pressures. Training must be relevant and respectful of their time. By listening and adjusting, we can support them better.

In the spirit of SDG-3 and WHO's Intersectoral Global Action Plan on Epilepsy and Other Neurological Disorders, we must act now. The window to build lasting systems for PCNS care and education is open. We must not lose it.

This chapter has explored challenges, solutions, and examples, but the journey is just beginning. We invite readers to take these ideas further. Apply them in your hospital, community, or classroom. Share what works. Learn from what does not. The path forward is one of cooperation, adaptation, and continued effort.

If we succeed, we will not only improve PCNS care. We will create systems that are smarter, more responsive, and more equitable, and we will do justice to those who have suffered in silence for too long.

Further Reading

1. Grisold W, Struhal W, Carroll WM, et al. The global burden of neurological disease: an urgent call to action. Lancet Neurol. 2022;21(5):389–90. https://doi.org/10.1016/S1474-4422(22)00110-5.
2. World Health Organization. Intersectoral global action plan on epilepsy and other neurological disorders 2022–2031. Geneva: WHO; 2022a. https://www.who.int/publications/i/item/9789240053690
3. World Federation of Neurology. Brain health: time matters in neurology. London: WFN; 2022. https://www.wfneurology.org/world-brain-day-202
4. Patel V, Saxena S, Lund C, et al. The lancet commission on global mental health and sustainable development. Lancet. 2018;392(10,157):1553–98. https://doi.org/10.1016/S0140-6736(18)31612-X.
5. Arora S, Thornton K, Murata G, et al. Outcomes of treatment for hepatitis C virus infection by primary care providers. N Engl J Med. 2011;364(23):2199–207. https://doi.org/10.1056/NEJMoa1009370.
6. Pakenham-Walsh N, Bukachi F. Information needs of health care workers in developing countries: a literature review with a focus on Africa. Hum Resour Health. 2009;7(1):30. https://doi.org/10.1186/1478-4491-7-30.
7. Reeves S, Pelone F, Harrison R, Goldman J, Zwarenstein M. Interprofessional collaboration to improve professional practice and healthcare outcomes. Cochrane Database Syst Rev. 2016;6:CD000072. https://doi.org/10.1002/14651858.CD000072.pub3.
8. Silverman J, Kurtz S, Draper J. Skills for communicating with patients. 3rd ed. CRC Press; 2013.
9. Kurtz SM, Silverman JD. The Calgary-Cambridge referenced observation guides: an aid to defining the curriculum and organizing the teaching in communication training programmes. Med Educ. 1996;30(2):83–9. https://doi.org/10.1111/j.1365-2923.1996.tb00724.x.
10. Oskoui M, Pringsheim T, Billinghurst L, et al. Practice guideline update summary: acute treatment of migraine in children and adolescents. Neurology. 2019;93(11):487–99. https://doi.org/10.1212/WNL.0000000000008095.
11. World Health Organization. Intersectoral global action plan on epilepsy and other neurological disorders 2022–2031. Geneva: WHO; 2022b. https://www.who.int/publications/i/item/9789240053694.

12. Wijeratne T, Crewther S. Post-COVID 19 neurological syndrome (PCNS); a novel syndrome with challenges for the global neurology community. J Neurol Sci. 2021;423:117329. https://doi.org/10.1016/j.jns.2021.117329.
13. Wijeratne T, Crewther SG. A systems neuroscience approach to diagnosis and rehabilitation of post COVID neurological syndrome based on the Systems Neuroscience Test Battery (SNTB) study protocol. NeuroRehabilitation. 2025;56(1):37–47. https://doi.org/10.1177/10538135241296773. Epub 2025 Apr 4. PMID: 40183164

Research Needs in Post-COVID Neurological Syndrome

8

Tissa Wijeratne and Sheila Crewther

8.1 Introduction—Rethinking Research for Post-COVID Neurological Syndrome

The COVID-19 pandemic has reshaped global health in ways no modern outbreak has done before. While the initial focus was understandably on acute infection and respiratory outcomes, attention has steadily shifted toward long-term sequelae, particularly the persistent neurological symptoms now recognized under the umbrella of Post-COVID Neurological Syndrome (PCNS) [10, 11]. These symptoms include brain fog, headaches, anosmia, paresthesia, mood disorders, cognitive dysfunction, autonomic disturbances, and fatigue, often affecting people well beyond their recovery from the acute phase [5]. PCNS does not follow a single trajectory [1–4]. Instead, it exhibits a broad clinical spectrum, variable duration, and no reliable biomarker or diagnostic tool. As a result, both diagnosis and treatment remain challenging. What has become clear is that we are facing not just a viral aftermath, but an entirely new dimension of chronic neurological disease that demands urgent scientific attention.

The current research landscape for PCNS is limited, scattered, and reactive. While some countries and institutions have launched studies to understand the phenomenon, these efforts often lack coordination, standardization, and translational scope. The World Health Organization has acknowledged the condition and called for global collaboration. Similarly, in Australia, the Parliament recently tabled submissions and expert hearings highlighting the gaps in care, research, and support for

T. Wijeratne (✉)
Department of Neurology and Stroke, La Trobe University, St. Albans, VIC, Australia
e-mail: tissa.wijeratne@wh.org.au

S. Crewther
Department of Neuroscience, La Trobe University, St Albans, Melbourne, VIC, Australia
e-mail: S.Crewther@latrobe.edu.au

T. Wijeratne, S. Crewther (eds.), *Post Covid-19 Neurological Syndrome*,
https://doi.org/10.1007/978-3-032-14995-4_8

individuals living with long COVID symptoms—including those with neurological manifestations. Despite these recognitions, sustained funding and structural research frameworks remain largely inadequate. A major concern is that the post-COVID condition has emerged into a health system already under strain, with limited bandwidth to take on yet another chronic disorder—especially one that challenges the boundaries between neurology, immunology, infectious disease, and mental health.

PCNS is not an isolated issue. Instead, it sits at the intersection of many overlapping scientific disciplines, requiring a fundamentally new research paradigm. The syndrome's varied and multisystemic presentation suggests that traditional, single-disease research approaches may not be sufficient. Investigations that narrowly focus on one pathway or organ system are unlikely to yield the integrated understanding necessary for diagnosis or therapy. Instead, a systems-level strategy is needed—one that maps the immune response, metabolic status, vascular injury, neural plasticity, and psychological resilience in a single framework. This shift requires not only new funding but also new mindsets, methodologies, and infrastructure.

Equally critical is the inclusion of diverse and representative populations. PCNS affects people of all ages, ethnicities, and pre-existing health statuses. Women appear disproportionately affected by long COVID, yet many existing studies are underpowered to explore sex-specific biological or psychosocial mechanisms. Likewise, marginalized populations, rural communities, and people with disabilities are often underrepresented in research despite being disproportionately affected by healthcare access barriers. Without inclusive research design, we risk developing interventions that fail to serve those who need them most.

Moreover, PCNS is emerging as a syndrome that could reshape how we think about post-viral illnesses more broadly. Many of its features resemble those seen in chronic fatigue syndrome (CFS/ME), post-concussive syndromes, and even autoimmune encephalopathies. If studied properly, PCNS could offer a unique window into understanding these historically misunderstood and under-researched conditions. It could also help reframe brain health research more broadly by bridging gaps between infectious triggers, chronic inflammation, neuroplasticity, and behavioral health. In short, PCNS represents not only a scientific puzzle but also an opportunity to build a more inclusive, holistic model for brain health research in the twenty-first century.

Technology, if used wisely, can accelerate this shift. Artificial intelligence (AI), especially in the form of explainable AI (XAI), offers tools to process high-volume, multi-dimensional data—exactly the type generated by PCNS patients undergoing blood biomarker testing, imaging, cognitive screening, and remote monitoring. Combined with wearable technologies, longitudinal real-world data, and structured patient-reported outcomes, AI can help identify disease patterns, predict risk trajectories, and propose personalized interventions. However, for AI to make a meaningful impact, it must be integrated from the ground up within ethical, transparent, and clinically grounded research frameworks. Smart, patient-centered data governance models must accompany these technologies to ensure trust and benefit sharing.

At the heart of this conversation is a broader shift in research values. PCNS research should not be driven solely by the availability of funding or the urgency of headlines. Instead, it should be grounded in the lived experience of patients, many of whom have become active participants, organizers, and even data scientists in their own right. Patient-led research collaborations have already produced some of the richest qualitative and epidemiological data on long COVID and PCNS. Their efforts must be elevated and integrated into mainstream research programs. Co-design, participatory science, and open-access data principles must form the bedrock of any meaningful PCNS research roadmap.

The need for standardized definitions and diagnostic criteria remains critical. While clinical case definitions have begun to take shape, there is still no global consensus on what constitutes PCNS versus other post-infectious or stress-related syndromes. Clearer case identification is essential not only for clinical trials but also for basic science investigations into mechanisms. Additionally, longitudinal cohorts must extend beyond a few months of follow-up. Many PCNS patients report symptom fluctuation or delayed onset, and only long-term studies will reveal whether we are dealing with self-limiting phenomena or chronic, lifelong conditions in certain subsets.

Lastly, research into PCNS must remain nimble and responsive. New SARS-CoV-2 variants, evolving vaccination patterns, reinfections, and shifting public health behaviors will all impact the natural history of PCNS. Research frameworks should be adaptable, with built-in mechanisms for rapid protocol updates, data harmonization, and international collaboration. This responsiveness will not only ensure the relevance of findings but also build resilience for studying future pandemics and their neurological consequences.

In this chapter, we explore these themes in greater detail. We outline the critical knowledge gaps, review current initiatives and their limitations, and propose a roadmap for future research. Our aim is to help build a research architecture that is inclusive, responsive, biologically informed, and grounded in lived experience. As PCNS continues to impact millions around the world, the scientific community must rise to meet the challenge, not only to understand this syndrome but to transform the way we think about brain health in the aftermath of infectious disease.

8.2 Recognizing the Urgency: A Systems Level Call to Action for Post-COVID Neurological Syndrome

Post-COVID Neurological Syndrome is emerging as one of the most urgent and complex challenges in contemporary brain health. What initially appeared as scattered and transient symptoms in some COVID survivors has now become a consistent and often disabling neurological condition affecting millions of people across all continents. The symptoms are diverse and persistent, including memory loss, slowed thinking, poor concentration, sleep disturbances, dizziness, sensory changes, autonomic dysfunction, and severe fatigue. These symptoms can last for months or even years after the initial infection and may significantly impair daily functioning, employment, and quality of life, yet the condition remains poorly understood, inconsistently identified, and often under acknowledged in clinical settings.

The scale and scope of this problem require a new way of thinking. We can no longer approach PCNS as a simple post viral complication. It is a complex disorder that affects the brain, immune system, metabolism, and vascular health simultaneously. These overlapping systems must be studied and treated together. A narrow or symptom focused approach will not be sufficient to address the full burden of the syndrome. The medical community must adopt a systems biology perspective, which considers the dynamic interactions between different organs, pathways, and environments in shaping health and disease.

A systems biology approach does not just mean collecting more data. It means asking better questions. What causes persistent inflammation in some patients but not in others? Why do some individuals develop severe cognitive issues while others experience mostly fatigue or dizziness? How do genetic, social, environmental, and psychological factors influence recovery? These are the questions that can only be answered through coordinated, multi dimensional research efforts that integrate molecular biology, clinical observations, digital health tools, and patient reported outcomes.

To truly understand and address PCNS, collaboration is essential. This must be a shared effort across many levels of care and inquiry. Researchers, public health experts, data scientists, and mental health professionals all have roles to play. Critically, the experience and insight of patients and caregivers must be at the center of this work. People living with PCNS are often the first to detect patterns, track symptoms, and trial interventions. Many are already contributing valuable data and participating in patient led research initiatives. Their knowledge is essential for identifying meaningful research questions, ensuring ethical study designs, and improving the relevance of findings.

Frontline clinicians, particularly general practitioners, neurologists, and rehabilitation specialists, are often the first point of contact for patients with PCNS. These professionals are witnessing the real world impact of the syndrome every day. They are also struggling with the lack of guidance, diagnostic tools, and treatment protocols to support patients effectively. Clinicians need tools that are both scientifically valid and practical to use in everyday care. This includes clear diagnostic frameworks, access to validated biomarkers, and referral pathways for complex cases. Training and support are also essential so that clinicians feel confident in managing this unfamiliar and evolving condition.

Despite growing awareness from national governments and global health bodies, funding and policy support for PCNS research remains far behind what is needed. Countries like Australia have begun to formally recognize the impact of long COVID and PCNS through parliamentary inquiries and public health strategies. The World Health Organization has published a clinical case definition and emphasized the importance of research coordination. These are critical steps. However, they must be matched with sustained investment in research infrastructure, equitable access to care, and the development of interdisciplinary teams who can lead innovative studies.

PCNS also highlights the need for new research cultures that break down traditional silos. Neurologists must work with immunologists. Psychologists must engage with geneticists. Clinicians must sit at the table with bioinformaticians, patient advocates, and policy makers. Only through this kind of connected thinking can we begin to map the full spectrum of PCNS and design interventions that are timely, tailored, and truly effective.

In short, we must act quickly, collaboratively, and intelligently. PCNS is not just a challenge for individual patients or single health systems. It is a global problem that reveals deeper limitations in how we currently study and treat complex neurological conditions. The time has come to rethink our models, include the voices of those most affected, and invest in a systems based approach that can turn knowledge into healing. This is not just a research need. It is a moral and clinical imperative.

Emerging data from large clinical cohorts make it increasingly clear that brain fog is one of the most persistent and disabling symptoms of Post COVID Neurological Syndrome [7]. A study by Nordvig and colleagues followed patients for a full year after COVID infection and found that nearly one in three continued to experience brain fog well after recovery from the acute illness. Importantly, this symptom was not associated with the severity of the initial infection, age, or preexisting health conditions. Instead, it was closely linked to other long COVID symptoms such as sleep disturbance, breathlessness, weakness, altered smell and taste, reduced activity, and overall poor perceived health. Brain fog was also significantly associated with social isolation, time off work, and lasting disability. These findings underscore that brain fog is not simply a vague or psychosomatic complaint. It reflects a deeper, biologically driven dysfunction that is yet to be fully explained. The fact that patients with mild or moderate acute illness can develop long-term cognitive impairment points to mechanisms beyond simple viral injury or oxygen deprivation. This calls for urgent investigation into neuroinflammatory responses, immune activation, and neural network disruption. Understanding the biology of brain fog is not just a research priority but a clinical necessity. Without a clearer picture of what drives this condition, effective treatments will remain out of reach, and millions will continue to suffer without answers.

As Emma Kavanagh has argued, "Neuroinflammation is a process triggered by an attack on the immune system [6]. Activation of microglia in response to an immune system challenge can lead to a significant impact on cognitive processes, such as learning, memory and emotional regulation." In the context of long COVID, persistent brain fog may be more than a symptom—it could be a manifestation of ongoing neuroimmune dysfunction. Inflammatory cytokines have been implicated in the suppression of neurogenesis, reduced synaptic plasticity, and changes in dendritic architecture, all of which are essential for healthy cognition. These biological disruptions are not fleeting events; they suggest a chronic alteration of brain function. This strengthens the case for long term, systems based research that tracks inflammatory markers, cognitive changes, and patient outcomes over months and years. Only through such sustained efforts can we begin to uncover how immune challenges evolve into chronic neurological syndromes. For conditions like Post COVID Neurological Syndrome, the urgency is clear: we must build longitudinal research frameworks that capture the full temporal and biological dimensions of this emerging disorder.

As Ali Nouraeinejad notes, there is growing evidence that individuals infected with COVID-19 face a high risk of developing long lasting neurological symptoms, most notably brain fog [8]. This cognitive dysfunction is increasingly recognized as a disabling feature of Post COVID Neurological Syndrome. While it was initially assumed that such outcomes would be limited to patients with severe disease, including those who required hospitalization or intubation, many individuals with mild or moderate infection and no hospital history are now reporting significant cognitive issues. These symptoms interfere with attention, memory, and executive function, and often persist for months. Brain fog significantly affects the ability to return to work, sustain social roles, and maintain a sense of wellbeing, yet despite its impact, the biological basis of brain fog remains largely unexplored. Understanding the mechanisms—whether they involve persistent inflammation, immune activation, microvascular injury, or disruptions to neurogenesis—is essential. It is not enough to acknowledge brain fog as a symptom. We must investigate it as a pathophysiological state. Targeted, biologically informed research is critical if we are to move toward accurate diagnosis, effective treatment, and meaningful support for those living with these cognitive burdens.

The urgency to move beyond symptom description toward actionable diagnostic and rehabilitation strategies for Post COVID Neurological Syndrome has never been greater. While brain fog and related symptoms have now been widely reported, the clinical community continues to lack standardized, scalable tools that can evaluate, monitor, and guide interventions for affected individuals. This is where the Systems Neuroscience Test Battery (SNTB) offers a timely and much-needed solution [9]. Developed by our group in response to the widespread and persistent neurological dysfunction seen in PCNS, the SNTB is designed as a rapid screening and evaluation framework grounded in systems neuroscience principles. It goes beyond isolated symptom tracking to explore how PCNS affects higher-order brain functions such as attention, perception, sensorimotor integration, and decision making—functions that are often impaired in patients reporting brain fog and cognitive fatigue.

The SNTB adopts a longitudinal, telehealth-enabled design that emphasizes accessibility, continuity, and objective measurement. It includes behaviorally relevant tasks that can be administered remotely, alongside structured assessments of clinical history, self-reported symptoms, neuropsychological function, and timed psychophysics. Critically, it incorporates visual and motor components to capture early signals of attention and coordination deficits, which often go undetected in routine clinical visits. By focusing on these foundational domains of brain function, the SNTB can help characterize the fluctuating and multisystem nature of PCNS with greater precision.

We offer this approach because existing diagnostic models are insufficient for the scope and complexity of PCNS. Standard cognitive tests are often too blunt to detect subtle dysfunctions in people with mild or moderate symptoms. At the same time, many patients struggle to access in-person clinics or specialists, especially those in rural or underserved regions. The SNTB's telehealth component directly addresses this barrier, providing a scalable and user-friendly platform that can be deployed in real-world settings with minimal burden to patients. This democratization of access is essential as the number of PCNS cases continues to grow globally.

Moreover, the SNTB integrates biological profiling to explore the underlying mechanisms of PCNS in a way that aligns with the systems biology approach we have long advocated. The study design includes paired radiological imaging and blood-based biomarker assessments to evaluate changes in brain structure, inflammation, and immune response over time. By synchronizing these datasets, we aim to identify both behavioral and molecular biomarkers that correlate with specific symptom clusters. This could ultimately support the development of targeted therapies and rehabilitation protocols tailored to the patient's unique biological and functional profile.

Another key advantage of the SNTB is its potential to guide and monitor rehabilitation. In addition to identifying deficits, the tool allows clinicians to track changes in function across repeated assessments, offering a real-time view of patient progress. This feedback loop can inform adaptive rehabilitation strategies, ensuring that interventions remain responsive to the evolving needs of the individual. Importantly, this approach supports shared decision making between clinicians, patients, and caregivers—building trust, transparency, and a clearer pathway to recovery.

The Systems Neuroscience Test Battery is more than a research protocol. It is a clinically grounded, patient-centered solution designed for the realities of modern medicine. It reflects our belief that managing PCNS requires more than isolated efforts. It demands a coordinated, systems-level approach involving neuroscience, immunology, digital health, and rehabilitation science, as well as the active participation of patients and frontline clinicians. By offering this tool, we aim to address a critical gap in PCNS care—one that continues to leave millions without answers or adequate support.

The time to act is now. As we continue to define the biological, cognitive, and emotional footprint of PCNS, tools like the SNTB will be central to the effort. They provide a way to move from observation to understanding, and from description to action.

8.3 Discussion

Post COVID Neurological Syndrome is not a rare complication—it is a widespread, disabling, and persistent disorder that continues to impact millions across the world. The symptoms, particularly cognitive dysfunction or "brain fog," are often invisible to standard medical investigations yet deeply disruptive to quality of life, employment, social engagement, and mental health. Despite these realities, our scientific understanding of PCNS remains fragmented. Clinical responses are often inconsistent. For frontline clinicians, managing PCNS means facing diagnostic uncertainty, patient distress, and a near total lack of evidence-based treatment pathways. For patients and caregivers, it often means months or years of being dismissed, misdiagnosed, or left without meaningful support.

What makes PCNS especially challenging is its systems-level nature. It cannot be understood by looking at a single organ, tissue, or symptom. Instead, it likely arises from a convergence of immune activation, neuroinflammation, autonomic imbalance, metabolic stress, and disrupted brain network function. The symptoms whether cognitive fatigue, post-exertional malaise, sensory sensitivity, or emotional dysregulation reflect underlying dysfunction in distributed brain systems. This points to the urgent need for a *systems biology approach* that captures the dynamic interplay between immune cells, cytokines, neurovascular function, brain connectivity, and behavior over time.

Systems biology offers a practical framework for decoding this complexity. Rather than isolating one biomarker or symptom, it enables integration. Blood-based inflammatory signatures, changes in brain structure and function on imaging, digital behavior tracking, and cognitive test scores can all contribute to a composite understanding of PCNS. This is particularly important for research, where overly narrow designs may miss the interconnectedness that defines the condition, but it is equally important for clinical care. If we can identify biological subtypes of PCNS such as a neuroinflammatory-dominant phenotype or an autonomic-dominant phenotype we can begin to personalize treatment, target rehabilitation, and reduce the burden of trial-and-error care.

Our proposed Systems Neuroscience Test Battery (SNTB) is designed with this in mind. It offers a structured, scalable, and clinically grounded way to assess PCNS in real-world settings. By combining timed psychophysics, neurocognitive tasks, telehealth delivery, and integration with biological sampling, the SNTB helps bridge the gap between clinical symptoms and systems-level insight. Critically, it supports longitudinal monitoring an essential aspect of PCNS research and care. Symptoms may fluctuate, relapse, or evolve over time. Single time-point assessments cannot capture the full disease trajectory. The SNTB enables repeated assessments that track progress, guide treatment response, and validate biological hypotheses through continuous patient engagement.

Equally vital is the role of *patient voices* in shaping this science. PCNS is one of the first large-scale neurological syndromes to emerge in the digital age with strong, coordinated patient advocacy. People living with long COVID have organized support groups, published qualitative data, participated in co-design, and actively shaped research agendas. This shift must not be reversed. In any meaningful PCNS research strategy, the involvement of patients and caregivers is essential—not as passive participants, but as equal partners. Their lived experience offers insights into symptom patterns, triggers, and treatment effects that no laboratory test can fully capture.

Incorporating *frontline clinicians* into the research framework is equally critical. General practitioners, emergency physicians, neurologists, and allied health professionals are seeing PCNS patients weekly, yet lack standardized tools, referrals, or training. Many clinicians express a sense of frustration and helplessness. Building PCNS research into clinical care pathways—through tools like SNTB or AI-driven symptom tracking—ensures that real-world expertise and patient complexity are not lost in translation. It also accelerates knowledge dissemination, as clinicians gain access to shared learning from emerging data.

The role of *explainable artificial intelligence (XAI)* in this context cannot be overstated. As we begin to amass large, complex datasets including biological samples, imaging, patient-reported outcomes, and wearable data AI becomes essential for pattern detection and risk modeling, but conventional black-box AI risks alienating clinicians and patients. Explainable models, by contrast, allow for transparency, trust, and collaborative interpretation. A model that shows why a patient is at high risk for prolonged brain fog highlighting elevated IL-6, reduced cognitive test speed, and disrupted sleep patterns provides a shared basis for discussion, planning, and care coordination. XAI also enables adaptive rehabilitation by predicting who may respond to which types of interventions based on multi-modal inputs.

For global policymakers and funding agencies, the emerging data on PCNS must serve as a wake-up call. This is not a rare condition. This is not limited to hospitalized patients. Brain fog, fatigue, dysautonomia, and cognitive instability are affecting a large percentage of working-age adults who were never admitted to hospital during their acute COVID infection. The economic, social, and healthcare burden of untreated PCNS is enormous. Without sustained research investment, workforce protection, and rehabilitation pathways, the long shadow of COVID-19 will continue for years, if not decades.

It is also important to acknowledge the *equity gap*. Marginalized populations, people with disabilities, those with limited access to care, and individuals in remote areas may face greater challenges in both the experience and diagnosis of PCNS. Telehealth tools like SNTB help close this gap by offering scalable and accessible diagnostics. But research must also address social determinants, language access, cultural safety, and policy barriers that affect equitable participation and outcomes.

Looking forward, PCNS research must embrace translational ambition. We need basic scientists, clinical researchers, data scientists, frontline health workers, patients, and public health officials to work together. Multi-center cohorts, standardized protocols, open data platforms, and globally aligned research priorities can speed discovery and implementation. As with stroke, cancer, and other complex syndromes, PCNS will benefit from a research ecosystem that moves from bench to bedside to community and back again.

In conclusion, PCNS represents a defining challenge and opportunity for modern neuroscience and public health. It forces us to confront the limits of traditional diagnostics, the fragmentation of post-infection care, and the deep need for integrated, human-centered science. By adopting systems neuroscience, explainable AI, participatory research, and tools like the SNTB, we take an essential step forward not only for PCNS, but for a new generation of science that listens to patients, respects complexity, and transforms care.

References

1. Chee YJ, Fan BE, Young BE, Dalan R, Lye DC. Clinical trials on the pharmacological treatment of long COVID: a systematic review. J Med Virol. 2023;95:e28289.
2. Chen Y, Allen AP, Fallon M, Mulryan N, McCallion P, McCarron M, Sheerin F. The challenges of mental health of staff working with people with intellectual disabilities during COVID-19–a systematic review. J Intellect Disabil. 2022;17446295221136231.
3. Choi UW, Ai X, Li H, Hao Y, Yao X, Guan Y. Immunosuppressive therapy and COVID-19 infection in patients with NMOSD. Immun Inflamm Dis. 2024;12:e1128.
4. Chow CP, Chesley CF, Ward M, Neergaard R, Prasad TV, Dress EM, Reagan S, Kalyani P, Smyk N, Turner AP, Agyekum RS, Ittner CAG, Sandsmark DK, Meyer NJ, Harhay MO, Kohn R, Auriemma CL. Patients' perspectives on life and recovery 1 year after COVID-19 hospitalization. J Gen Intern Med. 2023;38:2374–82.
5. Kaseka ML, Ly M, Yea C, Longoni G, Yeh EA. Impact of COVID-19 public health measures on myelin oligodendrocyte glycoprotein IgG-associated disorders in children. Mult Scler Relat Disord. 2021;56:103286.
6. Kavanagh E. Long Covid brain fog: a neuroinflammation phenomenon? Oxf Open Immunol. 2022;3.
7. Nordvig AS, Rajan M, Lau JD, Kingery JR, Mahmud M, Chiang GC, De Leon MJ, Goyal P. Brain fog in long COVID limits function and health status, independently of hospital severity and preexisting conditions. Front Neurol. 2023;14.
8. Nouraeinejad A. Brain fog as a long-term sequela of COVID-19. SN Comprehens Clin Med. 2022;5:9.
9. Wijeratne T, Crewther SG. A systems neuroscience approach to diagnosis and rehabilitation of post COVID neurological syndrome based on the Systems Neuroscience Test Battery (SNTB) study protocol. Neurorehabil Neural Repair. 2025;56:37–47.
10. Wijeratne T, Gillard Crewther S, Sales C, Karimi L. COVID-19 pathophysiology predicts that ischemic stroke occurrence is an expectation, not an exception-A systematic review. Front Neurol. 2020;11:607221.
11. Wijeratne T, Wijeratne C. Clinical utility of serial systemic immune inflammation indices (SSIIi) in the context of post covid-19 neurological syndrome (PCNS). J Neurol Sci. 2021;423:117356.

9 Therapeutic Options for Post-COVID 19 Neurological Syndrome

Reuben Parama Iswara and Tissa Wijeratne

9.1 Introduction

The COVID 19 pandemic has fundamentally altered the global health landscape. Beyond the acute respiratory illness that dominated early headlines, we are now facing the long tail of the pandemic. A significant proportion of individuals, many of whom had only mild initial illness continue to experience debilitating symptoms for months or even years. These individuals have often been grouped under the umbrella term "long COVID" or more formally, Post-Acute Sequelae of SARS CoV 2 infection (PASC).

But as we have argued throughout this book, this broad label hides more than it reveals. While long COVID encompasses a range of lingering symptoms across multiple organ systems, a striking majority by some estimates, close to 90% are neurological in nature. These include chronic fatigue, brain fog, memory issues, mood disturbances, dysautonomia, and sensory changes. This is not a footnote. This is the story. What we are witnessing is not a vague post-viral syndrome. It is a widespread, disabling neurological disorder. It is Post-COVID 19 Neurological Syndrome, PCNS.

Yet, despite the growing scale of this condition, we still have no established treatment guidelines. We have no universally accepted diagnostic criteria. We have no single pathway to care. This has led to enormous variability in how patients are managed, how clinicians interpret symptoms, and how researchers define outcomes. Without clear recognition of PCNS as a distinct neurological entity, treatment

R. Parama Iswara (✉)
Department of Neurology, Western Health, Melbourne, VIC, Australia
e-mail: Reuben.ParamaIswara@wh.org.au

T. Wijeratne
Department of Neurology and Stroke, La Trobe University, St. Albans, VIC, Australia
e-mail: tissa.wijeratne@wh.org.au

T. Wijeratne, S. Crewther (eds.), *Post Covid-19 Neurological Syndrome*,
https://doi.org/10.1007/978-3-032-14995-4_9

efforts remain scattered and reactive. We are trying to treat a condition we have yet to officially name.

This lack of clarity has real consequences. Patients are bounced between specialties. Clinicians are unsure whether they are dealing with psychiatric fallout, autonomic dysfunction, post-viral fatigue, or something else altogether. Research trials fail to enrol consistent populations. Funding is spread thinly across dozens of disconnected projects. What is needed now is a unified framework that recognises PCNS for what it is a multisystem neurological syndrome that requires a structured, collaborative approach to care and recovery.

The underlying mechanisms of PCNS are complex and still evolving, but one area of increasing interest is mitochondrial dysfunction. The mitochondria—those tiny powerhouses of our cells—play a central role in energy production, redox balance, immune regulation, and cellular signalling. When mitochondria falter, everything from fatigue to cognitive processing to immune function is affected. It is no surprise, then, that patients with PCNS often present with symptoms that mirror other mitochondrial and metabolic disorders.

Emerging research supports the link. Studies have shown that individuals with long COVID display markers of impaired mitochondrial respiration, increased oxidative stress, and altered energy metabolism. This may help explain the profound fatigue, poor exercise tolerance, and mental exhaustion reported by so many. In other post-infectious syndromes, including chronic fatigue syndrome and some viral encephalitides, similar mitochondrial signatures have been observed. PCNS appears to follow this pattern.

Understanding this link opens the door to new therapeutic options. If PCNS is, at least in part, a syndrome of disrupted energy metabolism, then interventions aimed at supporting mitochondrial function may hold promise. This includes pharmacological agents such as Coenzyme Q10, NAD+ precursors, antioxidants, and metabolic enhancers. It also includes non pharmacological strategies such as dietary modulation, exercise rehabilitation (appropriately titrated), stress management, and sleep restoration.

However, despite these promising leads, clinical trials remain scarce. Most interventions are being tried in isolation, in small cohorts, with inconsistent endpoints. This fragmented approach mirrors the early years of research into chronic fatigue syndrome and fibromyalgia, where lack of consensus and limited collaboration stalled progress. We must not repeat the same mistakes.

To move forward, we need multicenter collaborative trials. We need to agree on symptom clusters, functional endpoints, and biochemical markers. We need funding bodies to prioritize PCNS as a standalone neurological disorder worthy of urgent study. We need clinicians from neurology, rehabilitation, psychology, immunology, and primary care to work together. And most importantly, we need to listen to patients. Their lived experience must shape the research agenda and the care pathways we build.

In this chapter, we explore the therapeutic landscape of PCNS with honesty and urgency. We acknowledge what we know, what we are learning, and what remains uncertain. We review current pharmacological approaches, from antidepressants and anticonvulsants to anti inflammatories and supplements. We examine the role of cognitive rehabilitation, pacing strategies, physical therapy, autonomic rebalancing, and mindfulness-based interventions. We explore digital tools, peer support, and care coordination models, and we highlight experimental therapies currently under investigation.

But we do not just list options. We examine them in the context of a condition that is still being defined. We discuss their limitations. We identify gaps in the evidence. We question whether interventions tested in other conditions can be safely applied to PCNS, and we call for a shift from isolated fixes to comprehensive, personalized care.

We also highlight the risks of therapeutic nihilism. Too often, patients with PCNS are told that nothing can be done. Or worse, that it is all in their head. This attitude causes harm. It delays recovery. It drives people out of the workforce. It increases disability. It damages trust in the health system. While we may not yet have a magic bullet, there is much we can offer. Validation. Structure. Symptom relief. Hope. These are not minor outcomes. They are the foundation of care.

Finally, we set out a vision for future research. One that is inclusive. One that bridges basic science and bedside care. One that engages communities from both high and low income settings. One that uses accessible tools and open data. One that centers equity and diversity. PCNS affects women more than men. It affects people of color disproportionately. It affects those who were already living with disadvantage. These realities must be reflected in our research and in our treatment designs.

This chapter is not a final word. It is a call to action. The path ahead is challenging. But with the right framing, the right science, and the right partnerships, we can improve outcomes for people living with PCNS. We can turn scattered knowledge into targeted care, and we can begin to restore lives interrupted by a virus that continues to change the world.

The lack of clearly defined diagnostic criteria and structured treatment for Post-COVID 19 Neurological Syndrome (PCNS) has created not only a scientific gap but a serious ethical and human crisis. The scientific uncertainty has directly translated into patient marginalization. A powerful and timely study by Au et al. [2], published in *SSM Qualitative Research in Health*, captures this reality [2]. Surveying 334 long COVID patients in the United States, the researchers documented widespread accounts of dismissal, diagnostic delays, and the emotional harm caused when clinicians failed to validate patient experiences. Many respondents described these encounters as a form of "medical gaslighting"—being told their symptoms were imagined, stress-related, or not serious, despite significant functional impairment.

This phenomenon is global. We have observed the same pattern in Melbourne, Australia. Over the past three years, we have spoken with more than 1000 individuals living with PCNS as part of co-design workshops, patient listening sessions, and advocacy forums. These participants echoed the findings from Au et al.'s study almost verbatim. They described being disbelieved, bounced between specialists, or told to "wait it out." Many had exhausted their savings pursuing answers. Others gave up on seeking medical help entirely. The psychological toll of not being seen or heard especially when already living with debilitating symptoms was immense.

The root of this crisis lies in the fact that PCNS still lacks formal recognition as a distinct clinical entity. Instead, symptoms are often categorized under the broader term "long COVID" or the more academic "Post Acute Sequelae of SARS CoV 2 infection" (PASC). But as we have argued throughout this book, these terms are inadequate. They blur the lines between organ-specific damage, post-ICU syndromes, and what is clearly a unique and disabling neurological condition. Nearly 90% of people experiencing long COVID symptoms report signs consistent with PCNS, yet treatment remains generic, fragmented, and often dismissive.

What Au and colleagues highlight and what we have seen firsthand is that the struggle for effective treatment begins with the fight to be believed. This is not merely a clinical failure. It is what Au et al. describe as a form of "ontological politics". Patients are not just seeking care. They are seeking recognition that their reality is real. That their suffering is legitimate. When healthcare professionals fail to acknowledge this, they do more than deny care. They deny identity and agency.

Importantly, the burden of dismissal is not evenly shared. Gender, class, and racial inequalities all amplify these experiences. Women, in particular, have described being told their symptoms were due to stress, menopause, or anxiety. Migrant patients have reported language barriers compounding their frustration. Aboriginal and Torres Strait Islander communities face even greater hurdles to accessing neurologically informed care. In many cases, social determinants become clinical determinants.

As we discuss therapeutic options in this chapter, we must hold this context in mind. There is no effective treatment without trust. No recovery without recognition. If we fail to confront the structural and interpersonal dynamics that have sidelined PCNS patients, we will continue to offer piecemeal solutions to what is, at its core, a systemic failure. Multicenter clinical trials, inclusive care pathways, and genuine co-design with patients are not optional add-ons. They are the only way forward.

Patients living with PCNS are not only battling physical symptoms but are also navigating an overwhelming terrain of uncertainty. Thompson et al. [17] offer critical insights into this struggle through their longitudinal interviews with individuals experiencing long COVID [17]. The authors describe the condition as a "liminal state," where people are stuck between who they were before illness and who they are now becoming. These patients are not just trying to get better, they are trying to reclaim their identity in a world that no longer makes space for them. Many feel invisible in medical settings, uncertain in their social roles, and abandoned by a system that lacks both answers and compassion. Our own co-design workshops in Melbourne echoes this exact pattern. People told us they no longer recognized themselves, not just due to fatigue or memory loss, but because their sense of being a competent, connected person had fractured. These stories are not simply emotional they reflect the real and measurable damage that delayed diagnosis and lack of treatment causes. We must act now to address this dual crisis of biology and identity.

From a biological standpoint, mounting evidence suggests that PCNS is sustained by complex, ongoing disruptions to immune and metabolic systems.

Francavilla et al. [8] describe how "inflammaging" and "immunosenescence" conditions usually linked to ageing, are now appearing in people with post-COVID conditions [8]. This abnormal, chronic inflammation keeps the brain and body in a state of dysfunction. Current therapies, such as anti inflammatories and immunosuppressants, offer only partial relief. However, new classes of small molecules, including CB2 receptor agonists and formyl peptide receptor ligands, are showing promise in early studies. These are not fringe ideas. They are the next wave of targeted interventions that could restore balance to an immune system caught in overdrive. If we wait for perfect data before we act, we will fail a generation of patients who need help today. What is needed is bold investment in trials, collaborative testing of novel therapeutics, and a willingness to treat based on the best science available now, not after another decade of suffering.

Headaches are one of the most common and disabling symptoms experienced by people living with Post-COVID 19 Neurological Syndrome (PCNS). In a recent prospective cohort study, Ruhnau et al. [14] found that patients who developed new or worsened headaches after COVID 19 showed elevated levels of inflammatory markers such as CX3CL1, TGF-beta1, VEGF, and beta-NGF [14]. These molecules are not just academic findings, they are signals of an activated immune response in the brain, pointing specifically to microglial activation and peripheral sensitization. The data suggest that these post-COVID headaches are not simply stress related or a return of previous migraine. They represent a unique inflammatory process, possibly triggered by viral injury and sustained by immune dysfunction. The presence of such markers, even weeks after infection, adds weight to what many patients describe headaches (Post-Covid-19 Headaches) that feel different, more constant, and more resistant to usual treatment. These findings support a shift toward anti-inflammatory therapeutic strategies for headache in PCNS, especially in the early, subacute stages of illness when immune modulation may still be effective.

Beyond these immune markers, growing evidence also points to the involvement of neuropeptides such as substance P and calcitonin gene-related peptide (CGRP) in PCNS-related pain and headache syndromes [1, 12, 15]. Substance P drives neurogenic inflammation, promoting blood vessel permeability and amplifying pain pathways. CGRP is already known to play a central role in migraine, acting on blood vessels and sensory nerves to sustain chronic pain. There is reason to believe that both peptides are active in at least some PCNS subsets, particularly those with daily, migraine-like headaches or new facial pain syndromes. What is remarkable is that effective treatments already exist for these pathways. CGRP monoclonal antibodies and small molecule inhibitors have transformed migraine care in recent years. The question is—why have they not yet been tested in PCNS? These agents offer a potentially rapid and scalable solution, but clinical trials are urgently needed to evaluate their use in this context. PCNS is not one disease but a spectrum, and headache is often its earliest and most visible sign. The longer we wait, the more lives are disrupted, and the more entrenched these symptoms become. The tools are in our hands. It is time to use them wisely, guided by well-designed, inclusive, and collaborative research.

The recent review by Gheorghita et al. [9] reinforces the growing recognition that PCNS is a biologically complex condition with wide clinical variability [9]. Core symptoms such as cognitive slowing, fatigue, and persistent headaches reflect central nervous system dysfunction and are often shaped by factors like age, sex, comorbidities, and severity of the initial illness. The authors draw attention to chronic immune activation, vascular injury, and altered transcriptional pathways as key drivers of ongoing symptoms. These insights point to the need for targeted interventions, including anti-inflammatory therapies, neuroprotective agents, and metabolic support strategies.

While early, multidisciplinary rehabilitation remains important, it cannot be the only response. Structured cognitive and physical rehabilitation can improve function, but the underlying biology must be addressed to change disease course. Promising strategies including complementary therapies and lifestyle-based interventions require rigorous evaluation, particularly in resource-limited settings.

Ultimately, the path forward lies in deeper understanding and precise intervention. Inflammation, mitochondrial dysfunction, and inflammaging are not just theoretical constructs they are measurable, targetable processes. If we act now with well-designed clinical trials based on these mechanisms, we can move beyond symptom management toward meaningful recovery for people living with PCNS.

The review by Gupta et al. [10] underscores a critical but often overlooked dimension of Post-COVID-19 Neurological Syndrome its impact on children and adolescents. Drawing from 48 studies, the authors reveal that long COVID in young people includes both physical and neuropsychiatric symptoms, ranging from fatigue and sleep disturbances to anxiety, cognitive changes, and depression [10]. Some children also experience persistent neurological complaints even in the absence of a confirmed positive COVID test, suggesting that diagnostic limitations may obscure the true scale of the problem. While many symptoms resolve within six months, a concerning subset of children continues to experience functional impairments that disrupt learning, development, and daily life. The review also highlights the challenges of studying PCNS in paediatric populations, including heterogeneous symptom clusters and evolving diagnostic frameworks. Importantly, the authors call for multidisciplinary, holistic care that includes neurorehabilitation, psychological support, and close monitoring of school performance and social engagement. Long COVID in children is not a benign or rare phenomenon it is a growing issue with long-term consequences for mental health, education, and family wellbeing. These findings reinforce the urgent need for paediatric-specific clinical trials and early intervention strategies tailored to this vulnerable group.

Autonomic dysfunction is one of the most disabling yet under-recognized components of Post-COVID-19 Neurological Syndrome. Dotan et al. [7] highlight how SARS-CoV-2 may trigger autoimmune responses that target the autonomic nervous system, leading to symptoms such as fatigue, dizziness, heart rate variability, temperature dysregulation, and brain fog [7]. These symptoms mirror those seen in chronic fatigue syndrome and fibromyalgia, where dysautonomia is a key feature. What makes this especially concerning is the persistence of symptoms in otherwise healthy individuals, sometimes long after the acute infection has resolved.

Autoantibodies against G-protein-coupled receptors and renin-angiotensin system molecules have been implicated, suggesting an immune-mediated mechanism rather than just residual viral damage. Without targeted interventions, these autonomic disturbances can severely impair quality of life, limit physical activity, and fuel anxiety and depression. While immunotherapy such as IVIG or plasmapheresis may be warranted in select cases, non-invasive strategies like guided exercise therapy, hydration protocols, and autonomic rebalancing must be developed and tested in structured clinical trials. The nervous system does not recover passively in these cases active intervention is essential. Recognizing and treating dysautonomia is therefore central to any meaningful care pathway for PCNS.

The SingStrong programme offered a simple, non-pharmacological intervention that combines breathing retraining, mindfulness, and singing to address key symptoms of long COVID [4]. In this small pilot study, participants reported significant improvements in breathlessness, fatigue, voice quality, and cognitive symptoms after ten weeks of online sessions. The intervention was well tolerated, low cost, and accessible, making it a promising option for broader use. Importantly, some participants no longer met diagnostic criteria for chronic fatigue syndrome after the programme. While these early results are encouraging, larger, controlled studies are needed to confirm its effectiveness. Still, the SingStrong approach highlights how universally available tools like guided breathing and structured singing can support recovery and improve quality of life for people living with PCNS.

Fatigue remains one of the most persistent and disabling symptoms of Post-COVID-19 Neurological Syndrome, with few effective treatment options. A systematic review by Vollbracht and Kraft [18] explored the use of high-dose intravenous vitamin C in treating post-viral fatigue, including that associated with long COVID. Of the nine clinical studies reviewed, most reported significant reductions in fatigue levels, along with improvements in associated symptoms such as sleep disturbances, poor concentration, and low mood. The authors highlight that "oxidative stress, inflammation, and circulatory disorders" are key contributors to long COVID fatigue, and propose that the "antioxidant, anti-inflammatory, endothelial-restoring, and immunomodulatory effects" of vitamin C may offer therapeutic benefit. While further large-scale trials are required to confirm these findings, IV vitamin C appears to be a promising adjunct treatment, particularly in cases where fatigue is severe and functionally limiting. Its favorable safety profile and biological plausibility warrant closer investigation in PCNS-specific clinical trials.

Emerging evidence suggests that immune dysregulation plays a central role in the pathogenesis of PCNS, and targeted immunotherapy may offer relief for a subset of patients. In a small but compelling case series, Thompson et al. [16] reported significant improvements in six out of nine individuals with long COVID following long-term, high-dose intravenous immunoglobulin (IVIG) therapy [16]. These patients, who experienced symptoms lasting from 101 to over 500 days, presented with a combination of neurological, cardiological, and pulmonary issues common hallmarks of PCNS. All exhibited signs of immune perturbation, including suspected autoimmune activity, even though only one had a prior diagnosis of immunodeficiency. IVIG was administered over three months, and treatment continued in those showing clinical improvement. Notably, those who received the full course of therapy demonstrated either "significant" or "remarkable" benefit, reinforcing the potential of IVIG as a disease-modifying intervention in PCNS. While the study is limited by its small size and observational design, it adds to a growing body of literature suggesting that some long COVID symptoms may be driven by autoimmune or neuroinflammatory processes. Larger, controlled trials are urgently needed, but this report supports the rationale for testing immunoglobulin therapy in patients with persistent neurological symptoms, autonomic dysfunction, and biomarker evidence of immune activation.

Maladapted, chronic, low grade neuroinflammation is a likely core feature of Post-COVID-19 Neurological Syndrome and contributes to many of its most disabling symptoms, including anxiety, fatigue, cognitive fog, and persistent headaches. In a recent review, Cárdenas-Rodríguez et al. [5] explore the potential role of cannabinoids particularly cannabidiol (CBD), cannabigerol (CBG), and Delta-9-THC in modulating neuroimmune pathways relevant to PCNS [5]. These phytocannabinoids have demonstrated antioxidant, anti-inflammatory, and neuroprotective properties in other neurological and immune-mediated disorders. Given the overlap between neuroinflammatory cascades, cytokine dysregulation, and mood-related symptoms in PCNS, cannabinoids may offer dual benefits dampening inflammatory signals while alleviating anxiety and emotional distress. Importantly, this line of inquiry sits at the intersection of psychoneuroimmunology, highlighting how immune activity, psychological states, and neural function are deeply interwoven in post-viral syndromes. While promising, this approach requires careful validation. The review stresses the urgent need for well-designed, controlled clinical trials to assess the safety, efficacy, and optimal formulation of cannabinoid-based interventions in PCNS. These trials must also be equipped to measure outcomes beyond symptom severity, including quality of life, functional recovery, and biological markers of immune modulation. As we continue to uncover the pathways linking mind, brain, and immune system in PCNS, interventions targeting these psychoneuroimmunological axes should be a priority for future research.

A novel and unconventional window into patient experience with PCNS comes from an exploratory study by Bobak et al. [3], which analyzed Reddit posts discussing the use of psilocybin commonly referred to as "magic mushrooms" for treating neuropsychiatric symptoms of long COVID [3]. Of 110 posts meeting inclusion criteria, nearly 80% reported some level of symptom improvement, particularly in fatigue, cognitive fog, and depression. Notably, most of those who reported benefit experienced sustained improvement beyond the acute psychedelic experience, suggesting possible long-term modulation of brain function or mood. While anecdotal and drawn from self-reported online data, these findings reflect the growing interest in psychedelics as potential tools for treating neuroinflammatory and neuropsychiatric syndromes. They also point to a critical gap in current research: many people with PCNS are turning to unregulated, experimental self-treatments due to a lack of effective clinical options. This underscores the urgent need for carefully designed prospective studies to evaluate the safety, mechanisms, and therapeutic potential of psychedelics in PCNS. As we seek to understand the psychoneuroimmune underpinnings of long COVID, interventions like psilocybin may offer new pathways for symptom relief, but they must be explored within rigorous scientific and ethical frameworks.

As the neurological impact of long COVID becomes more evident, network-based approaches to drug repurposing offer a promising path forward. In a recent systems biology study, Qian et al. [13] constructed a comorbidity network linking COVID-19 with a range of central nervous system (CNS) disorders such as Alzheimer's disease, Parkinson's disease, multiple sclerosis, and autism spectrum disorder to identify overlapping molecular targets [13]. Using dynamic perturbation analysis and functional module detection, the authors identified a key pathway involving protein synthesis dysregulation and highlighted ubiquitin-carboxy-terminal hydrolase L1 as a novel target. Drug repurposing simulations suggested that compounds like pregnenolone a neurosteroid with known effects on cognition and inflammation could be potential therapeutic candidates for PCNS. This integrative framework supports the idea that PCNS shares common biological pathways with other neurodegenerative and neuroimmune conditions. Rather than starting from scratch, therapies developed for other CNS disorders may hold promise if strategically repurposed. However, these findings now require translation into in vivo and clinical research settings. Applying such network-based strategies to PCNS-specific datasets could accelerate discovery and help identify viable treatments faster, particularly in a landscape where traditional drug development timelines are too slow for the scale of patient need.

Hyperbaric oxygen therapy (HBO) is emerging as a promising, though still under-researched, intervention for the treatment of long COVID and its neurological manifestations. In their clinical review, Katz et al. [11] examined studies published between late 2021 and early 2024 and found that HBO delivered through controlled pressurized oxygen environments led to significant improvements in patients suffering from persistent post-COVID symptoms [11]. While the mechanism is still being investigated, HBO is believed to reduce neuroinflammation, improve mitochondrial function, and enhance oxygen delivery to damaged tissues, all of which are relevant to the pathophysiology of Post-COVID-19 Neurological Syndrome (PCNS). The therapy has shown benefit in case series and preliminary randomized trials, offering symptom relief in domains such as fatigue, cognitive impairment, and exercise intolerance. Given its established safety profile and biological plausibility, HBO stands out as a potential adjunctive treatment for PCNS. However, access, cost, and infrastructure remain significant barriers, and large, rigorously controlled clinical trials are urgently needed to confirm efficacy, optimize protocols, and determine which patient subgroups are most likely to benefit. As we search for scalable, mechanism-based interventions for PCNS, HBO represents a compelling option worthy of further exploration.

Low-dose naltrexone (LDN) has emerged as a potentially valuable intervention for some symptoms of Post-COVID-19 Neurological Syndrome (PCNS), but its role remains poorly understood and underexplored. While anecdotal reports and small-scale studies suggest possible benefits in managing fatigue, pain, and cognitive dysfunction symptoms commonly seen in PCNS—the biological mechanisms by which LDN exerts its effects are not yet well defined. It is thought to act through modulation of microglial activation and neuroinflammation, yet direct evidence in the context of long COVID is lacking. In their mini review, Dietz and Brondstater [6] highlight LDN, along with stellate ganglion block, as underutilized but potentially impactful therapies that warrant greater attention [6]. Despite its established safety profile and accessibility, there is an urgent need for controlled trials and mechanistic studies to validate its use in PCNS. Without clearer biological underpinnings, clinical application remains speculative. Future research should focus not only on efficacy but also on understanding how LDN interacts with the immune and nervous systems in post-viral conditions like long COVID. Until such data are available, LDN should be viewed as a promising candidate requiring further scientific validation not a substitute for evidence-based care.

Many patients in Melbourne have already begun accessing interventions such as low-dose naltrexone and stellate ganglion blocks through available integrative and interventional pain clinics. In our clinical observation, outcomes have been mixed some patients report meaningful improvements in fatigue, anxiety, and autonomic symptoms, while others experience minimal benefit. This variability underscores the need for more structured studies to identify which patient subgroups are most likely to respond and to better understand the timing, dosage, and mechanisms of action behind these therapies.

9.2 Discussion: The Path Forward for Therapeutic Research in Post-COVID-19 Neurological Syndrome (PCNS)

The therapeutic landscape for Post-COVID-19 Neurological Syndrome (PCNS) remains highly fragmented, despite growing recognition of its biological underpinnings and widespread impact. While numerous interventions—from neurorehabilitation to IVIG—have shown early promise, the evidence base remains weak, inconsistent, and often anecdotal. The urgent need for large-scale, collaborative, randomized controlled trials (RCTs) cannot be overstated. These trials must prioritize mechanistic precision, patient-centered outcomes, and real-world scalability. They should also move beyond siloed treatment arms to embrace integrated models that reflect the complexity of PCNS.

One key area that demands rigorous investigation is the use of nutraceuticals. Compounds such as curcumin, black pepper extract (piperine), Coenzyme Q10, taurine, and NAD+ precursors have demonstrated anti-inflammatory, antioxidant, and mitochondrial-supporting properties in related conditions. Given the evidence of mitochondrial dysfunction, oxidative stress, and immune dysregulation in PCNS, these agents are biologically plausible candidates for clinical trials. Curcumin, for example, inhibits key inflammatory pathways (e.g., NF-kB) and may reduce neuroinflammation, while piperine enhances its bioavailability. Coenzyme Q10 and taurine support mitochondrial energy metabolism and membrane stability, potentially improving fatigue and cognitive symptoms, yet these compounds remain relegated to the periphery of treatment strategies due to lack of formal study in PCNS cohorts.

Well-designed, placebo-controlled trials with biomarker integration could clarify their role and move them from theoretical to evidence-based care.

Simultaneously, pharmacological interventions targeting known inflammatory and neuropeptide pathways must be prioritized. The roles of calcitonin gene-related peptide (CGRP) and substance P in PCNS-related headaches, facial pain, and sensory dysregulation demand urgent attention. CGRP monoclonal antibodies and receptor antagonists have already revolutionized migraine treatment and are well tolerated. Their application in PCNS could offer rapid, targeted relief for a subgroup of patients experiencing daily, treatment-resistant headaches. Similarly, drugs modulating substance P pathways may help address chronic pain and neurogenic inflammation in PCNS subsets. These agents are ready for repurposing trials, and time should not be lost in initiating them.

Beyond these peptide-focused approaches, neuromodulation presents an exciting and underexplored frontier. Techniques such as transcranial magnetic stimulation (TMS), vagus nerve stimulation (VNS), and transcutaneous auricular stimulation may help recalibrate disrupted neuroimmune networks. Small studies have shown benefit in post-viral fatigue and depression—conditions that overlap substantially with PCNS. These modalities warrant inclusion in multidisciplinary trial platforms that can stratify patients by symptom cluster, autonomic function, and biomarker profile.

Psychiatric and psychoneuroimmunological symptoms of PCNS especially anxiety, depression, and dissociation should not be managed with default psychiatric labelling or isolated pharmacotherapy. Instead, they must be understood within the broader context of neuroinflammation and autonomic dysregulation. Trials assessing anxiolytic agents with dual immunomodulatory effects (e.g., SSRIs, SNRIs, low-dose atypical antipsychotics) should be coupled with measurement of inflammatory biomarkers, neuroimaging, and autonomic parameters. In parallel, non-pharmacological interventions like mindfulness-based stress reduction, cognitive behavioural therapy (CBT), and paced breathing should be incorporated into care pathways and rigorously tested in multicenter trials.

Cannabinoid-based therapies represent another promising domain. Cannabidiol (CBD) and related compounds exhibit anti-inflammatory, anxiolytic, and neuroprotective properties. Their potential role in modulating microglial activation, restoring immune balance, and alleviating neuropsychiatric symptoms warrants careful study. Randomized trials must move beyond recreational models to focus on standardized, pharmaceutical-grade preparations, optimal dosing regimens, and defined outcomes relevant to PCNS—including cognitive clarity, sleep quality, autonomic stability, and functional recovery.

Further still, the potential synergy between emerging immunotherapies and personalized medicine approaches should be explored. Immune surveillance tools such as cytokine panels, immune cell profiling, and gene expression assays may allow for stratification of patients into biologically meaningful subgroups. For instance, patients with persistent autoantibodies or evidence of immune exhaustion may benefit more from IVIG, plasmapheresis, or selective immunosuppressants. Others may respond better to metabolic and neuroplasticity-enhancing strategies. Such stratification must be embedded into trial design.

The growing public interest in psychedelic therapies, such as psilocybin, is another frontier worth examining with scientific rigour. The Reddit-based survey showing subjective improvement in fatigue, cognitive fog, and mood post-psilocybin use reflects unmet needs and patient desperation. These early signals should prompt pilot trials with appropriate ethical oversight and objective measurement tools to explore potential neuroimmune or neuroplastic benefits.

Equally important is the inclusion of hyperbaric oxygen therapy (HBO) in future research frameworks. By enhancing oxygenation, modulating inflammation, and potentially improving mitochondrial function, HBO aligns mechanistically with many of the biological disruptions seen in PCNS. Early studies and case reports are promising, but larger trials with sham control, neurocognitive endpoints, and inflammatory markers are needed.

Importantly, trials must also account for the accessibility, cost-effectiveness, and safety of interventions. Low-dose naltrexone (LDN), for example, has been used in various autoimmune and chronic pain conditions with minimal adverse effects. It may have a role in modulating microglial activity and immune tone in PCNS. However, mixed clinical outcomes in our own experience in Melbourne and the absence of mechanistic data underscore the need for controlled, biomarker-driven studies.

Collaborative research efforts should prioritize real-world implementation. This includes platform trials with multiple intervention arms, adaptive trial designs that allow for early signal detection, and embedding of trials within routine care settings such as long COVID clinics, rehabilitation centers, and primary care networks. Studies should also incorporate longitudinal follow-up to assess sustainability of benefits and delayed responses.

Finally, there is a critical need to include nutraceutical-pharmaceutical combination studies. For example, combining Coenzyme Q10 with a CGRP antagonist or curcumin with low-dose naltrexone may offer additive or synergistic benefits. These combinations must be grounded in biological plausibility, mechanistic rationale, and patient-centered outcomes.

In conclusion, we are standing at a turning point in PCNS therapeutics. The suffering is real, the biology is emerging, and the tools are within reach. What is missing is coordinated action. We must invest in high-quality, collaborative, multidisciplinary RCTs that not only test individual therapies, but also generate insights into the mechanisms, biomarkers, and care pathways that can guide a new era of personalized recovery. Anything less risks repeating the fragmented, ineffective approaches that have defined our response to other complex, post-infectious syndromes. The time to act is now.

References

1. Anichini A, Salvioni Chiabotti P, Bally J, Castro Jimenez M, Démonet JF, Di Virgilio G, Hirt L, Hottinger A, Kuntzer T, Michel P, Novy J, Pot Kreis C, Rossetti AO, Rouaud O, Théaudin M, Du Pasquier R. recent advances in neurology. Rev Med Suisse. 2021;17:196–200.
2. Au L, Capotescu C, Eyal G, Finestone G. Long covid and medical gaslighting: dismissal, delayed diagnosis, and deferred treatment. SSM Qual Res Health. 2022;2:100167.
3. Bobak L, Dorney I, Kovacevich A, Barnett BS. Therapeutic potential of psilocybin for treating neuropsychiatric long COVID symptoms: a reddit investigation. J Psychoactive Drugs. 2025:1–9.
4. Cahalan RM, Meade C, Mockler S. SingStrong-A singing and breathing retraining intervention for respiratory and other common symptoms of long COVID: a pilot study. Can J Respir Ther. 2022;58:20–7.
5. Cárdenas-Rodríguez N, Ignacio-Mejía I, Correa-Basurto J, Carrasco-Vargas H, Vargas-Hernández MA, Albores-Méndez EM, Mayen-Quinto RD, De La Paz-Valente R, Bandala C. Possible role of cannabis in the management of neuroinflammation in patients with post-COVID condition. Int J Mol Sci. 2024;25.
6. Dietz TK, Brondstater KN. Long COVID management: a mini review of current recommendations and underutilized modalities. Front Med (Lausanne). 2024;11:1430444.
7. Dotan A, David P, Arnheim D, Shoenfeld Y. The autonomic aspects of the post-COVID19 syndrome. Autoimmun Rev. 2022;21:103071.
8. Francavilla F, Intranuovo F, La Spada G, Lacivita E, Catto M, Graps EA, Altomare CD. Inflammaging and immunosenescence in the post-COVID era: small molecules, big challenges. ChemMedChem. 2025;20:e202400672.
9. Gheorghita R, Soldanescu I, Lobiuc A, Caliman Sturdza OA, Filip R, Constantinescu-Bercu A, Dimian M, Mangul S, Covasa M. The knowns and unknowns of long COVID-19: from mechanisms to therapeutical approaches. Front Immunol. 2024;15:1344086.
10. Gupta M, Gupta N, Esang M. Long COVID in children and adolescents. Prim Care Companion CNS Disord. 2022;24.
11. Katz AA, Wainwright S, Kelly MP, Albert P, Byrne R. Hyperbaric oxygen effectively addresses the pathophysiology of long COVID: clinical review. Front Med (Lausanne). 2024;11:1354088.
12. Pellesi L, Edvinsson L. Revisiting substance P in migraine: a methodological approach inspired by anti-CGRP and anti-PACAP success. J Headache Pain. 2025;26:22.
13. Qian J, Yang B, Wang S, Yuan S, Zhu W, Zhou Z, Zhang Y, Hu G. Drug repurposing for COVID-19 by constructing a comorbidity network with central nervous system disorders. Int J Mol Sci. 2024;25.
14. Ruhnau J, Blücher M, Bahlmann S, Zieme A, Vogelgesang A, Steinmetz A, Fleischmann R. Occurrence of new or more severe headaches following COVID-19 is associated with markers of microglial activation and peripheral sensitization: results from a prospective cohort study. J Headache Pain. 2024;25:101.
15. Schlereth T, Schukraft J, Krämer-Best HH, Geber C, Ackermann T, Birklein F. Interaction of calcitonin gene related peptide (CGRP) and substance P (SP) in human skin. Neuropeptides. 2016;59:57–62.
16. Thompson JS, Thornton AC, Ainger T, Garvy BA. Long-term high-dose immunoglobulin successfully treats Long COVID patients with pulmonary, neurologic, and cardiologic symptoms. Front Immunol. 2022;13:1033651.
17. Thompson CM, Gerlikovski E, Babu S, Mcguire M, Robieson I, Ranallo A. A longitudinal interview study of people with long COVID: uncertainties, liminality, and processes of becoming. Health Commun. 2024:1–12.
18. Vollbracht C, Kraft K. Feasibility of vitamin C in the treatment of post viral fatigue with focus on long COVID, based on a systematic review of IV vitamin C on fatigue. Nutrients. 2021;13.

Patient Needs in PCNS Care 10

Reuben Parama Iswara and Tissa Wijeratne

10.1 Introduction

From the earliest stages of the COVID-19 pandemic, voices in the neurological community warned of the potential for long-term sequelae affecting the brain and nervous system. Among them were Wijeratne and Crewther, who published in 2020 on the emerging evidence of neuroinvasion, immune dysfunction, and the likelihood of persistent neurological symptoms in the aftermath of SARS-CoV-2 infection [1–4]. Despite this foresight, systems failed to respond with the urgency or coordination required. Four years later, Post-COVID-19 Neurological Syndrome (PCNS) remains under-recognized, under-researched, and for many, untreated.

Part of the problem, as we have explored throughout this book, lies in the name. "Long COVID" is too vague, too generic, and too often dismissive of the neurological reality faced by the majority of sufferers. Nearly 90% of people with persistent post-COVID symptoms report issues related to the brain and nervous system—including cognitive dysfunction, fatigue, sensory changes, mood disturbance, and autonomic instability, yet the terminology has blurred clinical boundaries and diluted research efforts. In failing to name PCNS as a distinct condition, we have also failed to create pathways to care.

The Australian House of Representatives inquiry into long COVID, culminating in the 2023 report *Sick and Tired: Casting a Long Shadow*, laid bare the consequences of this inaction. It documented the testimonies of patients who had lost jobs, relationships, housing, and faith in the medical system. Many were women.

R. Parama Iswara (✉)
Department of Neurology, Western Health, Melbourne, VIC, Australia
e-mail: Reuben.ParamaIswara@wh.org.au

T. Wijeratne
Department of Neurology and Stroke, La Trobe University, St. Albans, VIC, Australia
e-mail: tissa.wijeratne@wh.org.au

T. Wijeratne, S. Crewther (eds.), *Post Covid-19 Neurological Syndrome*,
https://doi.org/10.1007/978-3-032-14995-4_10

Many were from culturally and linguistically diverse backgrounds. Many were young people who had previously been healthy. Their stories, woven throughout the report, reveal a health system caught off guard, underprepared, and slow to listen.

One patient recounted "I used to run every day. I haven't walked around the block in over a year. My GP told me to stop googling." Another described being told that her breathlessness and tremors were "anxiety-related," despite having no prior history of mental illness. These stories are not exceptions. They reflect a systemic pattern of diagnostic dismissal and therapeutic nihilism. As the report noted, "Patients reported repeatedly that they felt they were not believed."

This dismissal is not only emotionally damaging—it has measurable consequences. Delayed diagnosis leads to deterioration. Lack of recognition results in loss of services. The cumulative impact is one of despair. The Committee heard from parents of teenagers who had to leave school, from mid-career professionals forced into early retirement, and from regional patients who could not access specialists without driving hours while profoundly unwell.

Wijeratne and Crewther were not alone in sounding the alarm early, yet as the testimonies make clear, most patients felt abandoned. The report stated "Long COVID sufferers felt isolated in their illness, with little guidance on what to expect and few clinicians equipped to help." This gap between patient need and system response is the subject of this chapter.

We argue that addressing PCNS requires more than developing treatments. It demands a rethinking of how health systems validate, support, and walk alongside people living with complex, fluctuating neurological disability. That starts with recognition: not just naming PCNS, but recognizing its impacts across social, psychological, and economic domains.

Throughout this chapter, we draw on over 1000 lived experiences gathered through co-design workshops, listening forums, and advocacy collaborations across Australia. We explore what patients have told us they need—not just in terms of medication or therapy, but in terms of being heard, understood, and respected. We highlight the call for coordinated, multidisciplinary care and trauma-informed practice. We examine how social determinants intersect with clinical outcomes, and we present a roadmap for how health systems can shift from passive to proactive in supporting people with PCNS.

This is not just a medical challenge. It is a moral one. People with PCNS have been forced to prove their suffering, justify their symptoms, and fight for care. The time for disbelief is over. The time for system change is now.

In the sections that follow, we explore five domains of patient need:

1. Recognition and diagnostic legitimacy
2. Accessible and coordinated care pathways
3. Psychological and emotional support
4. Socioeconomic protection and workplace accommodations
5. Inclusion of lived experience in policy and research design

Each of these domains is informed by testimony, reinforced by evidence, and grounded in a vision of equitable, person-centered care. PCNS casts a long shadow, but with the right structures and values, we can begin to restore light.

10.2 Recognition and Diagnostic Legitimacy

At the heart of the crisis in Post-COVID-19 Neurological Syndrome (PCNS) care is the failure to formally recognize the condition. This lack of recognition affects every aspect of the patient journey, from how symptoms are interpreted to what treatments are offered and whether the illness is believed at all. Despite emerging as one of the most common and disabling manifestations of long COVID, PCNS remains poorly defined, inconsistently coded, and largely invisible in mainstream clinical practice.

Throughout the 2023 Australian parliamentary inquiry, the most consistent theme among patient testimonies was disbelief. People described being told they were exaggerating, misattributing their symptoms to anxiety, or simply overreacting. One participant testified, "It is hard enough not being able to remember my kids' names. But being told it is just stress almost broke me." For many, the denial of their symptoms by trusted professionals caused more harm than the symptoms themselves.

This is not a matter of semantics. Diagnostic labels carry real consequences. Without a recognized diagnosis, patients struggle to access income protection, disability supports, or specialist care. They are often ineligible for rehabilitation programs or excluded from clinical trials. Schools, employers, and insurance companies rely on coded conditions to validate absence or provide accommodations. When the label is missing or vague, so is the support.

A key finding from the inquiry was that the term "long COVID" itself has become a barrier to recognition. It is too broad and too easily dismissed. As several health professionals noted during hearings, it lacks specificity and diagnostic rigour. One clinician stated, "Long COVID is a bucket term. It is not a clinical entity in itself." This echoes what many patients have long felt that their neurological symptoms are qualitatively different and deserve their own category.

PCNS, by contrast, offers a clearer and more clinically grounded framework. It recognizes that neurological dysfunction including fatigue, brain fog, dysautonomia, and cognitive changes is not a footnote to long COVID but its central story. By naming PCNS explicitly, clinicians can begin to develop standardized pathways of care and guide appropriate referrals. Researchers can define inclusion criteria for trials. Health systems can monitor prevalence and plan services. Importantly, patients can receive validation and tailored care.

Wijeratne and Crewther called for this shift early in the pandemic. Their 2020 [1] and 2021 [3] commentaries emphasized the central role of neuroinflammation, mitochondrial dysfunction, and vascular injury in driving long-term symptoms. They urged health systems to adopt a syndromic approach one that connected the dots between immune activation and neurological outcomes. Unfortunately, these warnings were not widely heeded. The default remained reactive and reductive: treat the symptoms, not the system.

Changing this requires more than a new label. It demands education. Most general practitioners and emergency clinicians have had little to no training in recognizing PCNS. As a result, many default to psychiatric explanations or dismiss patients as difficult or demanding. This has eroded trust and led to harmful delays in diagnosis. Targeted education campaigns supported by clinical guidelines, coding reforms, and continuing professional development are urgently needed.

The report *Sick and Tired* recommended the development of clear diagnostic criteria and clinical definitions for long COVID subtypes, including those with predominantly neurological symptoms. This must be actioned as a priority. Diagnostic legitimacy will not come from patient stories alone, it will require institutional change and authoritative endorsement.

Medical colleges and specialty societies must also play a role. Neurologists, rehabilitation physicians, general practitioners, and allied health professionals all need clear guidance on how to identify PCNS, what investigations are appropriate, and what management strategies should follow. Shared decision-making, trauma-informed care, and continuity of care must be embedded from the outset.

Importantly, diagnostic legitimacy is not just about confirming a condition.it is about naming a reality. For many patients, getting a diagnosis is the first step in reclaiming control, understanding their bodies, and making informed choices. It is the beginning of recovery, even if treatment remains elusive.

One patient summed it up powerfully during the inquiry: "I can deal with being unwell. I just need to know that what I am experiencing is real and that someone else sees it too."

The health system must start seeing PCNS. It must start naming it, and it must start believing the people who live with it. Only then can we begin to repair the trust that has been so deeply damaged and create a foundation for effective care.

10.3 Accessible and Coordinated Care Pathways

Once recognition is achieved, the next critical challenge for patients with Post-COVID-19 Neurological Syndrome (PCNS) is accessing care that is timely, coordinated, and appropriately tailored. The current healthcare system in Australia, and in many other countries, is not designed to manage complex, fluctuating, multi-system syndromes. Patients with PCNS often find themselves navigating disconnected services, enduring long waits, and repeating their stories across multiple providers who may not speak to each other or share a unified treatment plan.

The 2023 parliamentary report *Sick and Tired: Casting a Long Shadow* was replete with examples of patients falling through the cracks. One woman described attending five different specialists over 12 months neurology, cardiology, psychology, respiratory, and infectious diseases without a single provider offering a unifying explanation for her symptoms or a lead role in coordinating her care. She said, "I felt like I was holding together my own medical file with duct tape."

This is not merely an issue of convenience. Lack of coordination leads to delays, duplication, conflicting advice, and ultimately poorer outcomes. For people with PCNS, whose symptoms may fluctuate dramatically over time, this inconsistency adds stress and undermines trust in the system. Worse still, some patients report being discharged from care entirely when their tests return normal, despite experiencing daily functional impairment.

Integrated care models must become the default approach for managing PCNS. This means establishing multidisciplinary teams where general practitioners, neurologists, rehabilitation specialists, psychologists, occupational therapists, and others work together under a shared framework. Such teams can coordinate diagnostics, streamline treatment plans, and provide holistic support across medical and psychosocial domains. Importantly, the patient must be at the center of this team—not passed between its edges.

Several countries have trialled specialist long COVID clinics with varying degrees of success. Australia's patchwork of services, however, remains highly variable by state and territory. Urban areas are more likely to have clinics linked to hospitals or university health networks, while rural and remote communities often rely on general practice alone. The inquiry heard from patients who travelled over 300 km to attend a single appointment, only to be told there was no further help available locally. Such disparities reinforce existing inequities in access to care.

Primary care plays a crucial role in any sustainable PCNS care model. However, general practitioners need support. They need clear guidelines, education on the neurological underpinnings of PCNS, and time to manage these complex cases. At present, many GPs report feeling overwhelmed, under-resourced, and unsure of where to refer. Introducing longer consultation items for PCNS, supported by Medicare, would be a strong step forward.

In our listening forums, patients emphasized the value of continuity and follow-up. Too often, care is transactional patients are seen once and discharged, with no plan for monitoring or adjustment. One participant shared, "I was told to come back if things got worse. I asked what that meant. The doctor just shrugged."

Care pathways must include routine follow-up appointments, proactive symptom monitoring, and access to case management. Case coordinators, particularly those trained in chronic disease management, can bridge the gap between primary and specialist care and ensure that patients are not left to manage alone. Digital tools, such as shared care plans and telehealth follow-ups, can enhance coordination especially for those in remote areas.

Mental health care must also be integrated, not siloed. Many patients with PCNS experience anxiety, depression, or trauma not as causes of their condition, but as consequences of prolonged illness, uncertainty, and dismissal, yet mental health services are often disconnected from neurological or rehabilitation care. A more compassionate, trauma-informed model would embed psychological support into the PCNS care pathway from the outset.

Equity must be central to any redesign. Aboriginal and Torres Strait Islander peoples, culturally and linguistically diverse communities, people with disability, and those with low health literacy are particularly vulnerable to fragmentation and under-service. Culturally safe care, interpreter services, outreach clinics, and community partnerships are essential to ensure that no one is left behind.

The report recommended the creation of a national clinical guideline for "long COVID care," which should include PCNS as a defined subtype. Ninety percent of long Covid is PCNS in our experience. This would provide consistency across jurisdictions and help align clinical training, service commissioning, and quality assurance. It would also enable evaluation and benchmarking of care models across states and territories.

The inquiry also called for the development of a national digital registry and a research and innovation fund for long COVID. These initiatives could support data-driven improvement in service delivery, enable real-time tracking of patient outcomes, and foster collaborative research into effective care models.

Finally, patients themselves must be included in the design and governance of PCNS services. Co-design is not just good policy it is essential for building trust, relevance, and responsiveness. Patients bring unique insight into what works and what does not. Their lived experience must shape everything from clinic hours to referral pathways, information materials, and research priorities.

As one patient stated during a co-design workshop in Melbourne, "We do not want pity. We want structure. We want someone to take responsibility for the journey not just tell us what door to knock on next."

PCNS requires a system-level response. It cannot be managed by piecemeal referrals or left to chance. Accessible, coordinated care pathways are not a luxury, they are a necessity. Without them, even the best intentions fall apart, but with them, we can begin to restore coherence, build trust, and support recovery in ways that are both clinically effective and humanly compassionate.

10.4 Psychological and Emotional Support

For many patients living with Post-COVID-19 Neurological Syndrome (PCNS), the most persistent and devastating impacts are not just physical. They are psychological, emotional, and existential. Across our listening forums, co-design workshops, and clinical encounters, a dominant theme has emerged: PCNS disrupts a person's sense of identity, safety, and belonging. The emotional toll of being sick for months or years without recognition, relief, or support is profound.

The parliamentary report *Sick and Tired: Casting a Long Shadow* captured this reality with striking clarity. Over and over, patients shared stories of fear, shame, grief, and a slow erosion of confidence. Many reported feeling trapped in a state of limbo, no longer able to fulfil their roles as parents, professionals, or community members. One participant said, "It feels like my body betrayed me, but worse like the world stopped believing I exist."

This is not an isolated experience. Mental health consequences of PCNS are widespread and well documented. Anxiety, depression, post-traumatic stress, emotional lability, and suicidal ideation are common and often directly linked to the illness experience, yet these symptoms are frequently misinterpreted as primary psychiatric conditions rather than secondary outcomes of chronic neurological illness. This misattribution is harmful. It leads to inappropriate treatment, delayed interventions, and a harmful narrative that blames patients for their own distress.

True psychological support for people with PCNS must begin with validation. That means recognizing the legitimacy of their illness and its psychological impact. It means believing patients when they say they are struggling not only with their bodies but with what their bodies are doing to their sense of self, future, and community.

In our Melbourne workshops, patients described the psychological experience of PCNS as a kind of exile. One woman in her early thirties said “I do not recognise my life anymore. I used to be strong and funny and confident. Now I plan my day around how much it will cost me to take a shower.” Another participant, a man in his forties, shared, “I know I look fine. That is the worst part. I am invisible in my suffering. People think I should be better by now.”

Psychological support, therefore, cannot be a late-stage add-on. It must be integrated into PCNS care from the beginning. Trauma-informed approaches are particularly important. Many patients report feeling retraumatized by their encounters with the healthcare system. Being dismissed, disbelieved, or gaslit has caused lasting psychological harm. Providers must be trained to approach patients with compassion, curiosity, and humility not defensiveness or suspicion.

This includes developing clinical environments where emotional expression is welcomed, not pathologized. It means asking not only “What is wrong?” but also “What has happened to you?” It involves validating the emotional consequences of being chronically unwell, isolated, financially strained, and socially disconnected.

Peer support programs can also play a critical role. Many patients report that the most healing conversations they have had were not with doctors or therapists, but with others living through similar experiences. Online forums, patient networks, and support groups provide validation, tips for coping, and a sense of community. However, these groups should not be seen as substitutes for professional care. Rather, they should be recognized, supported, and integrated into the broader ecosystem of recovery.

Access to mental health care remains a significant barrier for many patients. Waitlists are long, costs are high, and many providers lack knowledge of PCNS. In some cases, patients are referred to mental health professionals as a way of deflecting their physical symptoms, not addressing their emotional needs. This undermines trust and may deter patients from seeking support again.

The solution lies in embedding psychological services within PCNS care models. This includes routine screening for mental health concerns, on-site or telehealth access to psychologists and counsellors, and training for all clinicians in basic mental health first aid and communication skills. Funding models must allow for longer appointments, multidisciplinary case conferencing, and non-stigmatizing language.

The emotional burden of PCNS extends beyond the individual. Families, carers, and loved ones often experience secondary trauma, stress, and burnout. Partners may have to take on caregiving roles, parents may lose income or stability, and children may struggle to understand the changes in their family dynamics. These ripple effects must be acknowledged and supported. Family-inclusive care models and carer-specific resources are urgently needed.

One carer told us, "I am not just looking after my partner. I am trying to keep our family together while pretending everything is normal. But nothing is normal. And I do not know how long we can keep this up."

For young people with PCNS, the psychological impact can be particularly disorienting. Adolescents and young adults are in critical stages of identity formation, social development, and educational achievement. A sudden and prolonged illness at this stage can derail future plans and lead to long-term psychological scars. Schools, universities, and youth services must be brought into the care conversation. Flexible learning plans, counselling support, and advocacy services can help mitigate long-term impacts.

Culturally responsive care is also vital. Different communities understand and express emotional distress in different ways. Mental health services must be linguistically appropriate, culturally safe, and free from assumptions about what distress looks like. Interpreter services, peer navigators, and partnerships with community health organizations can help bridge these gaps.

10.5 Socioeconomic Protection and Workplace Accommodations

The economic and occupational consequences of Post-COVID-19 Neurological Syndrome (PCNS) are as devastating as the clinical and emotional ones. The condition strikes individuals across all age groups, backgrounds, and levels of previous health, but its persistence often forces people out of work, reduces household incomes, disrupts careers, and pushes many to the economic brink. Despite this, systems of social protection and workplace policy have been slow to adapt.

The *Sick and Tired* report includes testimony from countless individuals who could no longer maintain employment due to fatigue, brain fog, dysautonomia, or sensory overload. One respondent wrote, "I was told to try part-time work. I tried. After two hours, I could not remember my own password. I cried for a week. I have never felt so ashamed."

This shame is not inherent to illness. It is a symptom of societal failure. When people are punished for being unwell or forced to pretend to be well to survive, the system is broken. The experience of economic abandonment compounds the trauma of the illness itself. Many patients described being denied income support, rejected by insurers, or pressured to return to work before they were physically or cognitively ready. Others recounted long and demoralizing assessments by job service agencies that did not understand PCNS and treated them as malingerers.

We must fundamentally rethink the systems designed to protect individuals during times of health crisis. This begins with formally recognizing PCNS as a disabling condition under employment law and social protection frameworks. Until this occurs, people with PCNS will continue to fall through administrative gaps. Without diagnostic legitimacy and official coding, many are unable to access income protection, disability support, workplace leave entitlements, or superannuation access. This is particularly true for casual workers, contractors, or those in precarious employment.

The situation is even more acute for women, who make up the majority of PCNS sufferers and are often in caregiving roles or part-time employment. One mother shared, "I had to quit my job to look after my teenager who cannot get out of bed. Now we have no income and I am told I need to be job seeking or I will lose our payments."

This intersection of gender, caregiving, and chronic illness must be central to any policy response. Governments must implement gender-sensitive policies that account for both direct and indirect PCNS disability. Carers need targeted support, and households affected by PCNS should be eligible for hardship relief packages, rental support, and energy subsidies.

Workplace accommodations must also become more flexible and inclusive. Employers need education on PCNS. Many managers and HR departments have never heard of the condition or believe it is psychosomatic. Employees report being disbelieved, subjected to disciplinary procedures, or denied reasonable adjustments. In some cases, employees were told to get a note from a specialist, despite long waiting lists or no access to one at all. Others were offered a fixed return-to-work plan that did not account for fluctuating symptoms.

What is needed is a flexible, person-centered approach. This could include variable working hours, task modification, extended recovery time, assistive technology, and hybrid or remote working options. Most importantly, the individual should be consulted and empowered to shape a plan that suits their needs. One size does not fit all. Just as symptoms vary, so too do capacities and needs.

Occupational physicians, rehabilitation specialists, and vocational support workers must be brought into the conversation early. Workplace accommodations are most successful when coordinated by professionals who understand both the condition and the demands of the job. This requires workforce training and the development of clinical return-to-work guidelines specific to PCNS.

Governments can play a leading role. They should invest in pilot programs that partner healthcare services with employment support agencies. These models, which have been trialled for mental health and disability programs, could be adapted for PCNS. Support packages could include case coordination, workplace advocacy, and phased return-to-work programs with income subsidies for employers.

One innovation worth exploring is the concept of a "recovery wage" a guaranteed basic income for those who are unable to return to work but are not yet permanently disabled. This recognises the fluctuating nature of PCNS and allows people to focus on recovery without the constant pressure to prove their worthiness for support. It also reduces the long-term burden on the health system by preventing relapses and worsening illness due to economic stress.

Insurance providers must also update their frameworks. Many policies rely on outdated criteria for disability that do not account for neurological fatigue, cognitive impairment, or invisible symptoms. Reform is needed to ensure that PCNS sufferers are not excluded from coverage based on criteria that do not reflect the condition's realities. Regulatory oversight is needed to enforce fair assessment processes, appeal rights, and transparent decision-making.

Education systems also need reform. Students with PCNS report being forced to withdraw from study, denied special consideration, or placed under unrealistic performance expectations. Schools, TAFEs, and universities must develop protocols for accommodating students with PCNS. This includes flexibility with attendance, assessment deadlines, and alternative learning arrangements. Guidance counsellors and disability officers must receive training to support these students without stigma or scepticism.

The same applies to medical and allied health students. Those affected by PCNS may face both health and reputational risks, especially when their peers or faculty do not recognize the condition. The academic and clinical placement systems must ensure equity and reasonable adjustments for PCNS-affected trainees.

Housing security is another urgent issue. Patients reported losing rental properties due to loss of income, being unable to pay mortgages, or moving in with family in overcrowded and unstable conditions. Some became homeless. Housing assistance programs must include PCNS in their eligibility criteria. Public housing waitlists should prioritize individuals whose housing instability is tied to long-term post-viral disability.

People with PCNS also face challenges navigating legal systems. Some lose custody arrangements, are denied access to insurance claims, or struggle to obtain guardianship for dependents due to their illness. Legal aid services and community legal centers must be resourced to provide support for this emerging group. Policymakers should also consider appointing a dedicated PCNS ombudsman to oversee complaints related to systemic neglect, access barriers, or discrimination.

Social stigma remains a major barrier. Many patients are told they are lazy, dramatic, or faking. This stigma compounds economic hardship by making it harder to ask for help or advocate for oneself. Public education campaigns can help shift the narrative. Just as stigma around mental illness has slowly changed, so too must our understanding of invisible neurological illness. PCNS is real. It is disabling, and it deserves to be treated with compassion and dignity.

Finally, lived experience must shape socioeconomic policy. Governments and employers should create advisory councils that include patients, carers, clinicians, and economists. These councils can co-design programs, monitor their implementation, and ensure that funding is directed where it matters most. Policy must be grounded in reality not abstract economic models.

As one patient said in their submission to the inquiry, "I have lost my health, my job, my home, and my independence. But what hurts most is losing my dignity. Please help us get that back."

We owe it to them to do better. Socioeconomic protection and workplace accommodations are not separate from health. They are health. Without them, recovery is impossible. With them, we can build a more just and resilient system for all.

10.6 Inclusion of Lived Experience in Policy and Research Design

No meaningful reform in the care of people living with Post-COVID-19 Neurological Syndrome (PCNS) can occur without the genuine inclusion of those who have lived it. From health service design to policy development and clinical research, the voices of patients and carers must be placed not at the margins, but at the center. It is not enough to consult them. They must be recognized as experts in their own right experts in survival, navigation, adaptation, and resilience.

This principle is reinforced repeatedly throughout the 2023 Australian parliamentary inquiry report *Sick and Tired: Casting a Long Shadow*. Time and again, the Committee heard that patients were not just struggling with their symptoms they were battling a system that seemed determined to exclude them from decision-making. As one witness said, "We are not data points. We are living this. Let us be part of the solution."

Lived experience offers irreplaceable insights. Patients know where the care gaps lie. They know which services are helpful and which are harmful. They understand the nuanced ways symptoms affect daily function. They can see, often more clearly than clinicians or policymakers, how systems fail to connect and how language can wound or heal.

This chapter is informed by over 1000 conversations with PCNS patients across Australia. These individuals participated in co-design forums, workshops, listening sessions, and surveys led by academic, advocacy, and community groups. Their reflections shaped the priorities, tone, and direction of this work. Their frustrations, insights, and solutions are not merely anecdotes. They are data—rich, grounded, and urgently relevant.

What patients want, above all, is to be believed and involved. In many cases, individuals with PCNS are already generating solutions: peer support groups, symptom tracking apps, guides for navigating healthcare appointments, and informal networks that share everything from treatment experiences to emotional support. These grassroots innovations often arise in the absence of formal support. Rather than ignoring or competing with them, the system should learn from and support them.

One of the clearest lessons from the inquiry was that systems designed without patients tend to serve bureaucracy, not healing. Eligibility criteria, referral pathways, appointment structures, and even clinic environments often reflect institutional convenience rather than patient needs. This mismatch erodes trust. When people feel invisible in systems that are meant to help them, disengagement follows. For PCNS, where patient fatigue and cognitive burden are already high, navigating disconnected or inflexible systems becomes an additional health threat.

Genuine co-design changes this. It moves from asking patients to provide feedback after the fact, to involving them in the creation of systems from the beginning. It requires cultural humility, shared language, transparent processes, and respect for different forms of knowledge. Importantly, co-design must include people from diverse backgrounds, including First Nations communities, people with disability, young people, migrants, and rural residents.

Researchers must also embed lived experience at every stage of study design. This includes setting priorities, developing research questions, determining inclusion criteria, shaping data collection tools, and interpreting results. Funding bodies should mandate lived experience involvement in all PCNS-related grants and provide resources to support it. Advisory boards should include patient representatives with decision-making authority, not symbolic roles.

At present, many patients feel research is done “on them” rather than “with them.” They are rarely told the outcomes of the studies they participate in. Their contributions are often unpaid. This must change. Compensation for time, expertise, and emotional labor is not just ethical—it is essential for equity. Researchers should also commit to accessible dissemination of results, including plain language summaries, multilingual translations, and formats accessible to people with fatigue or cognitive impairment.

One promising model is the Patient-Led Research Collaborative, a global group of long COVID patients who conduct and publish peer-reviewed research grounded in their collective experiences. Their work has significantly influenced the global understanding of post-COVID conditions and highlights what is possible when lived experience is placed at the forefront.

Australia should support the development of similar structures, including national patient-led PCNS research hubs and partnerships with academic institutions. These hubs can collect data, generate insights, and evaluate services in ways that are both rigorous and grounded. They can also act as accountability mechanisms, ensuring that policies and practices align with the realities of those affected.

Policy design must follow the same logic. Whether at the national, state, or local level, PCNS-related programs and funding decisions must be shaped by those with firsthand experience. Governments should establish PCNS advisory panels composed primarily of people living with the condition, supported by carers, clinicians, and advocates. These panels should have real influence over how funding is allocated, how services are delivered, and how success is measured.

Metrics of success must shift. Too often, systems evaluate programs based on efficiency or throughput, not on whether patients feel better, more supported, or more in control. Lived experience perspectives can help design outcome measures that reflect what truly matters: the ability to manage daily life, to feel safe in healthcare settings, to be seen as a whole person.

Education and training are another key domain. Lived experience should inform the development of curricula for health professionals, especially in general practice, allied health, and emergency settings. Training should include real patient stories, co-facilitated teaching, and reflection on implicit biases. This helps build empathy, reduce stigma, and improve clinical care.

Digital health and artificial intelligence tools must also reflect lived experience insights. If telehealth platforms, symptom trackers, or clinical decision support tools are not designed with cognitive fatigue or fluctuating symptoms in mind, they risk excluding the very people they are intended to help. Accessibility must be a foundational design principle, not an afterthought.

Lived experience inclusion is not just about equity, it is about effectiveness. When patients are partners, the system works better. When their insights shape services, outcomes improve. When their realities guide research, the findings are more relevant. When their needs are centered in policy, justice becomes possible.

One patient said, “We have become the case managers of our own condition, the data analysts of our own symptoms, the advocates of our own rights. All we ask is to be recognized as what we already are experts.”

As this chapter closes, it is worth remembering that inclusion is not an endpoint. It is an ongoing practice. It asks systems to listen, to share power, and to reflect on their assumptions. It asks professionals to move beyond diagnosis to dialogue. It asks all of us to see each other, fully and respectfully.

PCNS will continue to challenge our health systems, research institutions, and policy structures, but it also offers an opportunity, a chance to build more human, more responsive, and more just systems. If we accept the leadership of those living with PCNS, that opportunity can become reality.

10.7 Discussion and Conclusion

One of the co-authors of this chapter recently reviewed a 46-year-old woman living with Post-COVID-19 Neurological Syndrome (PCNS). By the time she arrived in our clinic, she had already accessed nine different allied health providers and had been seen at a “Long COVID clinic” supported by a national Medical Research Future Fund (MRFF) grant. She was prescribed eleven medications to manage her symptoms, many in dangerously high doses. One antihistamine was prescribed at twelve times the recommended level, despite there being no published evidence to support its use for long COVID. After six months of intensive intervention, she had experienced no improvement. Her condition had not changed, but her trust in medicine had eroded. The first and most important task in her recovery was to begin the careful weaning off medications that had offered no benefit and, in some cases, may have caused harm.

This single case, although extreme, reflects a broader truth about PCNS. When systems fail to name the condition correctly, they also fail to treat it appropriately. The result is often a well-funded and well-meaning avalanche of disjointed care that burdens rather than supports. What the patient needed, like so many others, was not a list of speculative treatments but a clear, compassionate framework. She needed someone to name her condition as PCNS, to explain the current limits of knowledge honestly, and to work alongside her in building a personalized plan rooted in support, pacing, and safety. Most of all, she needed a care team committed to doing no harm.

Throughout this chapter, we have outlined the needs of people living with PCNS across five key domains: diagnostic legitimacy, coordinated care, psychological support, socioeconomic protection, and the inclusion of lived experience. The testimony from hundreds of individuals across Australia tells us the same thing: PCNS is real, it is disabling, and it is being overlooked. Too many people have suffered silently or been mislabelled with anxiety, conversion disorders, or lifestyle issues. Too many have been forced into fragmented systems that cannot see the full picture.

The first task must be recognition. PCNS is a distinct neurological condition, emerging with identifiable biological mechanisms, a consistent clinical profile, and profound personal and societal impacts. Naming it clearly is not just about semantics, it is about justice, resource allocation, and care design. Only when the condition is recognized can the system begin to respond in a coherent and meaningful way.

Equally important is the principle of informed care. Patients must be kept informed every step of the way—about what is known, what is uncertain, and what is possible. Clinical teams must resist the pressure to over-treat or rush to unproven protocols. The mantra should be listen first, inform clearly, and intervene cautiously. PCNS management is not a race to the most aggressive therapy. It is a long-term partnership built on trust, communication, and shared goals.

In the rush to respond to long COVID, there is a risk of repeating the same mistakes that have historically marginalized people with chronic, post-viral conditions. Many of the people now being labelled as "long COVID patients" have clinical presentations nearly identical to those with myalgic encephalomyelitis, post-viral dysautonomia, or complex fatigue syndromes. We must honour this history, not erase it. The insights from decades of lived experience with these conditions should be integrated into every policy and program we develop for PCNS.

We also must reject false binaries. PCNS is not either neurological or psychological. It is not either real or invisible. It is not either treatable or untreatable. It is a condition that exists in complexity, and our systems must evolve to meet that complexity with humility and integrity. That means multidisciplinary care. It means embedding mental health support in every care pathway. It means building economic safety nets that recognize fluctuating disability, and it means empowering patients to help lead the way.

There is hope in this story. The advocacy of patients, the growing body of research, the acknowledgement of PCNS in parliamentary and policy discussions, all of these are signs of progress. This book itself is a testament to the power of collaboration, cooperation, and communication. It has been shaped by neurologists, patients, researchers, policy experts, and community leaders working together. It reflects a shared commitment to listening, learning, and improving.

PCNS presents one of the most urgent and defining health challenges of our time, but it is also an opportunity a chance to rethink how we care, how we listen, and how we build. If we embrace that opportunity with clarity and courage, we can move from fragmentation to coordination, from dismissal to dignity, and from silence to shared purpose.

We invite our colleagues across all sectors, clinical, academic, community, and governmental to join us in this effort. Let this be the beginning of a new era of patient-informed, equity-driven, and evidence-based care. Together, we can chart a better path forward.

References

1. Wijeratne T, Crewther S. Post-COVID 19 Neurological Syndrome (PCNS); a novel syndrome with challenges for the global neurology community. J Neurol Sci. 2020;419:117179.
2. Wijeratne T, Crewther SG. A Systems neuroscience approach to diagnosis and rehabilitation of post COVID neurological syndrome based on the systems neuroscience test battery (SNTB) study protocol. NeuroRehabilitation. 2025;56:37–47.
3. Wijeratne T, Wijeratne C. Clinical utility of serial systemic immune inflammation indices (SSIIi) in the context of post covid-19 neurological syndrome (PCNS). J Neurol Sci. 2021;423:117356.
4. Wijeratne T, Gillard Crewther S, Sales C, Karimi L. COVID-19 pathophysiology predicts that ischemic stroke occurrence is an expectation, not an exception – a systematic review. Front Neurol. 2020;11:607221.

11 Brain Fog in the Young Insights from a Meta-analytic Review of Cognitive Impairment in Pediatric PCNS

Melanie J. Murphy, Lauren Falcone, and Nina Riddell

11.1 Introduction

Post-COVID Neurological Syndrome (PCNS) refers to persistent brain-related symptoms after COVID-19. These symptoms are common in adults and older adults recovering from the infection [5, 8, 9, 13]. But growing reports suggest that children may also be affected (e.g., [17, 23, 35]).

While the impact of PCNS in adults is becoming clearer, far less is known about how children are affected. Children are often thought to recover quickly from COVID-19. However, new evidence shows that a proportion of children continue to experience symptoms long after the infection ends. Prevalence estimates of PASC in pediatric populations vary greatly, with reports ranging from <10% to >60% [30, 40]. PASC in in children is often characterized by PCNS symptoms such as problems with concentration, forgetfulness, and general confusion [3, 4]. In some studies, up to half of children report trouble focusing, and many continued to have problems months after infection [3]. Cognitive assessments conducted in hospital settings have found measurable impairments in attention, memory, and executive functions—skills that are essential for planning, time management, and task completion. For example, Gonzalez-Aumatell et al. [17] reported that 60% of children attending a long-COVID unit screened against the Pediatric Symptom Checklist (PSC) screening tool were shown to exhibit cognitive dysfunction in areas such as attention (approximately 60%) and executive function (approximately 50%), and information processing speed (approximately 30%) after more intensive neuropsychological assessment. These difficulties can affect day-to-day functioning, making it harder for children to learn, keep up at school, and connect socially with peers

M. J. Murphy (✉) · L. Falcone · N. Riddell
School of Psychology and Public Health, La Trobe University, Melbourne, VIC, Australia
e-mail: m.murphy@latrobe.edu.au; l.falcone@student.unimelb.edu.au; n.riddell@latrobe.edu.au

T. Wijeratne, S. Crewther (eds.), *Post Covid-19 Neurological Syndrome*, https://doi.org/10.1007/978-3-032-14995-4_11

[17]. As childhood and adolescence are critical times for brain maturation, any disruption to typical developmental periods, especially in the acquisition of cognitive skills such as attention and memory, will have lasting effects across the lifespan.

Despite such concerns, there is a notable gap in understanding how widespread and pervasive these problems are, and how different aspects of cognition in children are affected following COVID infection. Thus, our team conducted a systematic review and meta-analysis to address this issue to characterize the common cognitive problems exhibited by children with PASC, and to define the domains of cognitive functioning impacted by the condition.

11.2 Methods

This review followed the PRISMA 2020 guidelines to ensure quality and transparency. It was registered in advance with the Open Science Framework in May 2024 (DOI: 10.17605/OSF.IO/7SC4M).

To find relevant studies on cognitive problems in children after COVID-19, we searched four major databases: PubMed, Ovid Medline, Ovid Embase, and Web of Science. The final search was completed in November 2024. The search strategy combined terms related to COVID-19, cognition, and young people. It included various ways of referring to COVID-19 (e.g., "long COVID," "PASC," "SARS-CoV-2"), cognitive functioning (e.g., "cognitive," "neuropsychological"), and age groups (e.g., "child," "adolescent," "teen"). The search was limited to studies published in English since 2020.

Search results were screened using Covidence software [39]. To be included, studies had to, be original, peer-reviewed, and published in English after January 2020, include participants under 18 years of age who had COVID-19 and met their country's definition of Post-Acute Sequelae of COVID-19 (PASC), use validated cognitive assessments; either performance-based tests or self/parent reports, and include children who were or were not hospitalized. For each included study, we recorded key information including the publication details, participant demographics, how long after infection testing occurred, hospitalization and symptom severity, and the type of cognitive tests used. We assessed the quality of each study using the Joanna Briggs Institute checklist for cross-sectional studies [25] to determine the risk of bias.

For the main analysis we used DSM-5 cognitive domains (e.g., complex attention, learning and memory) to group results and identify the proportion of children showing clinically significant cognitive impairment. Meta-analyses were conducted using the jamovi MAJOR module (Version 1.2.4). We calculated pooled prevalence estimates of cognitive impairment using arcsine transformation to stabilize variance. Heterogeneity was assessed using the I^2 and τ^2 statistics [19, 33]. Publication bias was examined using Kendall's tau [16]. For studies that could not be included in the meta-analysis, we presented a narrative synthesis. Where possible, we calculated Hedges' g to compare cognitive outcomes between PASC and control groups.

This approach provided both quantitative and qualitative insights into the prevalence and severity of cognitive problems in pediatric PCNS.

11.3 Findings and Interpretation

11.3.1 Prevalence of Cognitive Impairments in Pediatric PASC

Complex Attention Our meta-analysis shows that clinically significant cognitive impairments are common in children with Post-COVID Neurological Syndrome (PCNS) (Fig. 11.1) [12]. The most frequently affected domain was complex attention, with approximately half of the children showing clinically significant or at-risk levels of impairment. This aligns with what we know from adult PCNS research, where attention deficits are also prominent [6, 7]. Attention difficulties in children often impact learning, memory, and problem-solving, creating a cascade of effects impacting academic performance, even on a daily basis [27, 31]. Importantly, this was observed not only in formal psychometric tests but also in parent and self-reports [3, 4, 37].

Learning and Memory Memory and learning problems were also highly prevalent (42% of cases). Children with PCNS frequently struggled to retain new information, follow instructions, or complete tasks—a pattern also seen in adult PASC studies [13, 17]. One study included in our review [35] showed higher rates of memory impairment among hospitalized children, suggesting that symptom severity may increase cognitive risk. This mirrors adult findings linking more severe illness to worse neurocognitive outcomes [5, 24].

Working Memory and Executive Function Approximately 42% of pediatric PCNS patients also had impairments in working memory and executive function. These issues may present as difficulty remembering instructions, solving maths problems, planning tasks, or regulating emotions [11]. While the risk of publication

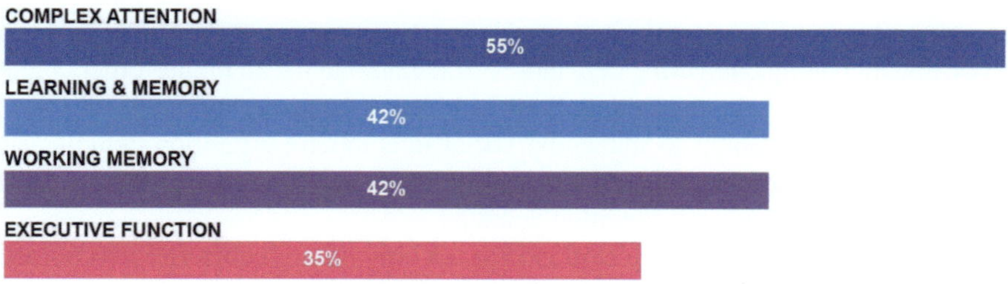

Fig. 11.1 Percentage of pediatric PASC patients showing clinically significant impairment, or significant risk of impairment in different cognitive domains

bias in these domains was high, the observed patterns still reflect known symptom clusters across age groups [17, 28, 32].

Narrative Synthesis and Additional Insights Studies not included in the meta-analysis supported the same trends. Children with PCNS performed worse on executive function tasks than controls who apparently had not been infected with COVID-19. The deficits were greater in those who were hospitalized, suggesting a dose-response relationship between infection severity and cognitive impact [15]. Interestingly, some moderate effect sizes were also observed in the verbal comprehension domain, despite insufficient data to include it in meta-analysis.

11.4 Theoretical and Clinical Implications

The findings from this systematic review and meta-analysis reinforce a growing body of evidence that PCNS significantly affects cognitive function in children. While much of the early literature has focused on adult populations, our study confirms that children are also susceptible to the long-term consequences of SARS-CoV-2 infection. PCNS is not solely a medical issue; it is also a neurocognitive one, with profound implications for health, development and education.

In classrooms, children may be mislabelled inattentive, unmotivated, or behaviorally difficult, when these issues are a consequence of post-viral cognitive fatigue or executive dysfunction. Teachers, school psychologists, and pediatricians need greater awareness and clear, practical guidelines to identify and support children experiencing PCNS appropriately.

At a systems level, this review highlights the need to screen pediatric COVID-19 patients for cognitive changes especially those with hospitalization, fatigue, or persistent physical symptoms. Health systems must integrate neuropsychological follow-up into pediatric COVID care pathways.

11.4.1 Complex Attention as a Core Deficit

The most consistent and concerning finding is the high prevalence of impairment in complex attention. This domain, responsible for sustaining focus, switching between tasks, and managing competing demands, is foundational for all higher-order cognitive activity [27, 36]. In children, deficits here can affect every aspect of life; from learning in the classroom to managing social interactions. Attention deficits also compromise the encoding of new information into memory, creating a cascade of dysfunction across multiple cognitive domains.

Importantly, these deficits were identified not only through objective psychometric tests but also through parent and self-reports, highlighting that children and caregivers themselves perceive the burden of PCNS deficits on cognitive function in daily life. While formal testing remains the gold standard for clinical diagnosis, caregiver input provides valuable early warning signs and can inform school-based accommodations. The findings highlight an urgent need for the development of validated, age-appropriate, rapid screening tools that can be used in schools, primary care, and outpatient settings to detect cognitive difficulties as soon as possible.

11.4.2 The Role of Memory and Executive Function

Closely linked to attention, impairments in learning, memory, and executive function were also highly prevalent. These functions facilitate information processing, planning, behavioural regulation, and emotional control. Executive dysfunction in children may present as impulsivity, emotional outbursts, or difficulty completing multi-step tasks; symptoms that are often misinterpreted as behavioural issues [11]. In classroom environments, this may lead to children being defined as displaying problematic or disruptive behaviours, when in reality they are experiencing executive dysfunction arising stemming from immunologically induced "brain fog" [10]. Without thorough assessment, children with PCNS risk being misdiagnosed or receiving interventions that fail to address the underlying cognitive impairment.

11.4.3 Dose-Response and Risk Stratification

The infection dose-response relationship observed in studies where hospitalized children exhibited greater cognitive impairment than non-hospitalized peers is particularly noteworthy. This pattern suggests that COVID-19 severity may be directly linked to long-term neurocognitive outcomes. It also strengthens the case for neuropsychological screening as part of routine discharge planning for children hospitalized with COVID-19, or those reporting persistent symptoms during recovery.

This review underscores the need to screen pediatric COVID-19 patients for cognitive changes, particularly those with a history of hospitalization, chronic fatigue, or persistent physical symptoms. Health systems must integrate neuropsychological follow-up into pediatric COVID care pathways to ensure early identification and intervention. These cognitive domains are foundational skills for healthy development and academic achievement. Left unaddressed, impairments can have enduring consequences.

11.4.4 Parallels with CFS/ME and a Systems-Based View

The similarities between PCNS and Chronic Fatigue Syndrome/Myalgic Encephalomyelitis (CFS/ME) are striking and informative. Both conditions involve persistent fatigue, cognitive dysfunction, and immune dysregulation [21]. While PCNS patients may show slightly less attentional dysfunction than those with CFS/ME, the symptom overlap is sufficient to support the use of shared screening tools, such as the DePaul Symptom Questionnaire [21]. This cross-condition perspective advocates for a systems-based approach to PCNS, viewing it not merely as a post-viral consequence but as part of a broader neuroinflammatory syndrome.

Such an approach also acknowledges that vaccination, though critical for reducing acute disease severity, may not entirely prevent cognitive impairment [26]. Thus the possibility of PCNS complications should not be dismissed in fully vaccinated patients, particularly in vulnerable populations such as those described above. This raises critical questions about individual susceptibility, immune resilience, and the role of repeated infections. Future research must prioritize studies that stratify children by vaccination status, prior health history, and socio-environmental context to better understand these trajectories.

11.4.5 Limitations and Gaps in the Literature

Despite the consistency of core findings, several limitations must be acknowledged. Only a small number of studies met the inclusion criteria for meta-analysis, limiting statistical power. Most studies lacked key demographic data such as ethnicity, socioeconomic background, or vaccination history, making it difficult to explore how these factors influence cognitive risk. Sex- and age-related differences, including distinctions between children and adolescents, could not be reliably analyzed due to insufficient reporting.

While most studies employed valid tools, methodological variation in sample size, design, and assessment strategy contributed to significant variability in the data. Moreover, the concentration of studies in high-income countries, particularly the USA and Italy, limits the global applicability of the findings. Cultural, educational, and healthcare differences across regions may affect both the expression and detection of PCNS.

Crucially, data on several cognitive domains (for example, language, perceptual-motor function, and social cognition) were lacking. These areas, which also depend heavily on intact attention and memory [14, 18], are likely affected but remain under-investigated. Future research must broaden its scope to build a more comprehensive picture of the neurodevelopmental impact of PCNS.

11.4.6 Educational and Clinical Implications

The educational implications of these findings cannot be overstated. Many children with PCNS will struggle in school, not due to a lack of motivation or intelligence, but because of subtle or moderate cognitive impairments affecting processing speed, working memory, or executive function. Without adequate teacher training and school-based support systems, these children risk academic underperformance, disengagement, and mental health complications.

The findings also point to an urgent need for multidisciplinary follow-up care. Pediatricians, neurologists, psychologists, and educators must work collaboratively to design care pathways that recognize cognitive impairment early and deliver tailored interventions. Delays in support may have lifelong developmental consequences, particularly for younger children whose neural systems are still in critical phases of maturation.

11.4.7 Standardizing Post-COVID Cognitive Screening

At present, there is no international consensus on screening for or managing cognitive impairment in children post-COVID. This represents a major oversight in pandemic recovery planning. The findings call for the development of international guidelines that include:

- Consensus definitions of pediatric PCNS-related cognitive impairment
- Standardized, age-sensitive neurocognitive screening protocols
- Inclusion of parent and teacher-reported measures to provide ecological validity
- Training modules for general practitioners, pediatricians, and educational psychologists

Given the overlap with ME/CFS and other inflammatory syndromes, existing interventions warrant exploration in the context of PCNS. Preliminary evidence from related conditions suggests these strategies may have the potential to improve function and quality of life [20, 22, 34], but further investigation is urgently needed to confirm.

11.4.8 Understanding the Whole Child

A final, essential consideration is the need to view children with PCNS holistically. Cognitive deficits often do not occur in isolation. Many children also experience sleep disturbances, anxiety, autonomic symptoms, or chronic fatigue [2, 17, 29]. These multifaceted presentations require a comprehensive, child-centred approach that considers emotional wellbeing, social functioning, and family dynamics alongside cognitive recovery.

Anecdotal evidence from families and clinicians suggests that without early and coordinated support, children may experience school absence, peer withdrawal, and developmental regression. These outcomes are especially concerning for children from marginalized or low-income communities, who already face systemic barriers to healthcare and education.

11.5 Conclusion

In summary, this review reveals a consistent and troubling pattern: cognitive impairments, particularly in attention, memory, and executive function, are common in children with Post-Acute Sequalae of Covid-19 (PASC). These domains are essential for learning, emotional regulation, and social engagement. The long-term consequences of these impairments extend beyond the clinic into classrooms, homes, and communities.

The findings call for a paradigm shift in how we understand and address pediatric COVID recovery. PASC is not only a respiratory or fatigue-based syndrome, but also a significant neuroimmunologically associated neurocognitive disorder that demands sustained attention from health, education, and policy sectors. Early screening, appropriate diagnosis, and multidisciplinary interventions must become standard components of pediatric COVID care.

We hope this chapter creates the impetus towards broader attention to the long-term neurological effects of COVID-19 in children. With timely screening, informed intervention, and coordinated care, we can mitigate the risk of enduring cognitive deficits and support optimal developmental trajectories for affected children to help prevent long-term harm.

We urge national and international health authorities to incorporate PCNS into COVID recovery frameworks. Clinicians must be trained to recognize and manage cognitive symptoms; schools must be equipped with the resources and guidance to support affected students; and researchers must invest in longitudinal studies to understand the natural history, treatment response, and psychosocial impact of PCNS.

As we transition into the next stage of pandemic response, the goal must be to prevent a silent epidemic of cognitive disability in children. This will require new tools, coordinated services, and a commitment to leaving no child behind. With early recognition, compassion, and evidence-based care, we can reduce suffering, preserve developmental potential, and help these children return to a trajectory of healthy growth and learning. The challenge is urgent, but solvable.

Acknowledgements We thank Dr. Hayley Pickering for her support in mapping neuropsychological assessments to DSM-5 cognitive domains.

References

1. American Psychiatric Association. Diagnostic and statistical manual of mental disorders. 5th ed; 2013. https://doi.org/10.1176/appi.books.9780890425596.
2. Basaca D-G, Jugănaru I, Belei O, Nicoară D-M, Asproniu R, Stoicescu ER, Mărginean O. Long COVID in children and adolescents: mechanisms, symptoms, and long-term impact on health – a comprehensive review. J Clin Med. 2025;14(2):378.
3. Brackel CLH, Lap CR, Buddingh EP, van Houten MA, van der Sande L, Langereis EJ, Bannier M, Pijnenburg MWH, Hashimoto S, Terheggen-Lagro SWJ. Pediatric long-COVID: an overlooked phenomenon? Pediatr Pulmonol. 2021;56(8):2495–502. https://doi.org/10.1002/ppul.25521.
4. Buonsenso D, Munblit D, De Rose C, Sinatti D, Ricchiuto A, Carfi A, Valentini P. Preliminary evidence on long COVID in children. Acta Paediatr. 2021;110(7):2208–11. https://doi.org/10.1111/apa.15870.
5. Ceban F, Ling S, Lui LMW, Lee Y, Gill H, Teopiz KM, Rodrigues NB, Subramaniapillai M, Di Vincenzo JD, Cao B, Lin K, Mansur RB, Ho RC, Rosenblat JD, Miskowiak KW, Vinberg

M, Maletic V, McIntyre RS. Fatigue and cognitive impairment in Post-COVID-19 Syndrome: a systematic review and meta-analysis. Brain Behav Immun. 2022;101:93–135. https://doi.org/10.1016/j.bbi.2021.12.020.

6. Cerioli M, Giacovelli L, Nostro C, Larini L, Castiglioni M, Scarpa C, Cassina N, Nicotra A, Maestri G, Cucumo V, Masserini F, Pomati S, Cirnigliaro G, Pantoni L, Dell'Osso B. Post-COVID condition: a focus on psychiatric symptoms and diagnoses in patients with cognitive complaints. CNS Spectr. 2024;1–7 https://doi.org/10.1017/S1092852924000464.
7. Charles James J, Schulze H, Siems N, Prehn C, Quast DR, Trampe N, Gold R, Faissner S. Neurological post-COVID syndrome is associated with substantial impairment of verbal short-term and working memory. Sci Rep. 2025;15(1):1695.
8. Chen C, Haupert SR, Zimmermann L, Shi X, Fritsche LG, Mukherjee B. Global prevalence of post-coronavirus disease 2019 (COVID-19) condition or long COVID: a meta-analysis and systematic review. J Infect Dis. 2022;226(9):1593–607. https://doi.org/10.1093/infdis/jiac136.
9. Delgado-Alonso C, Diez-Cirarda M, Pagan J, Perez-Izquierdo C, Oliver-Mas S, Fernandez-Romero L, Martinez-Petit A, Valles-Salgado M, Gil-Moreno MJ, Yus M, Matias-Guiu J, Ayala JL, Matias-Guiu JA. Unraveling brain fog in post-COVID syndrome: relationship between subjective cognitive complaints and cognitive function, fatigue, and neuropsychiatric symptoms. Eur J Neurol. 2025;32(1):e16084. https://doi.org/10.1111/ene.16084.
10. Denno P, Zhao S, Husain M, Hampshire A. Defining brain fog across medical conditions. Trends Neurosci. 2025;48(5):330–48. https://doi.org/10.1016/j.tins.2025.01.003.
11. Diamond A. Executive functions. Annu Rev Psychol. 2013;64(1):135–68.
12. Falcone L, Riddell N, Murphy MJ. Cognitive Impairment in Paediatric PCNS: a systematic review and meta-analysis. medRxiv. 2025; https://doi.org/10.1101/2025.05.29.25328543.
13. Fanshawe JB, Sargent BF, Badenoch JB, Saini A, Watson CJ, Pokrovskaya A, Aniwattanapong D, Conti I, Nye C, Burchill E, Hussain ZU, Said K, Kuhoga E, Tharmaratnam K, Pendered S, Mbwele B, Taquet M, Wood GK, Rogers JP, Leek CE. Cognitive domains affected post-COVID-19; a systematic review and meta-analysis. Eur J Neurol. 2024;32(1):e16181. https://doi.org/10.1111/ene.16181.
14. Fisher AV. Selective sustained attention: a developmental foundation for cognition. Curr Opin Psychol. 2019;29:248–53. https://doi.org/10.1016/j.copsyc.2019.06.002.
15. Frolli A, Ricci MC, Di Carmine F, Lombardi A, Bosco A, Saviano E, Franzese L. The impact of COVID-19 on cognitive development and executive functioning in adolescents: a first exploratory investigation. Brain Sci. 2021;11(9) https://doi.org/10.3390/brainsci11091222.
16. Gjerdevik M, Heuch I. Improving the error rates of the Begg and Mazumdar test for publication bias in fixed effects meta-analysis. BMC Med Res Methodol. 2014;14:109. https://doi.org/10.1186/1471-2288-14-109.
17. Gonzalez-Aumatell A, Bovo MV, Carreras-Abad C, Cuso-Perez S, Domenech Marsal E, Coll-Fernandez R, Goicoechea Calvo A, Giralt-Lopez M, Ensenat Cantallops A, Moron-Lopez S, Martinez-Picado J, Sol Ventura P, Rodrigo C, Mendez Hernandez M. Social, academic, and health status impact of long COVID on children and young people: an observational, descriptive, and longitudinal Cohort Study. Children (Basel). 2022;9(11) https://doi.org/10.3390/children9111677.
18. Harvey PD. Domains of cognition and their assessment. Dialog Clin Neurosci. 2019;21(3):227–37.
19. Higgins JPT, Eldridge S, Li T. Including variants on randomized trials. In: Higgins JPT, Thomas J, Chandler J, Cumpston M, Li T, Page MJ, Welch VA, editors. Cochrane handbook for systematic reviews of interventions. Cochrane; 2019. https://training.cochrane.org/handbook.
20. Hsu C-Y, Ahmad I, Maya RW, Abass MA, Gupta J, Singh A, Joshi KK, Premkumar J, Sahoo S, Khosravi M. The potential therapeutic approaches targeting gut health in myalgic encephalomyelitis/chronic fatigue syndrome (ME/CFS): a narrative review. J Transl Med. 2025;23(1):1–21.
21. Jason LA, Johnson M, Torres C. Pediatric post-acute sequelae of SARS-CoV-2 infection. Fatigue. 2023;11(2–4):55–65. https://doi.org/10.1080/21641846.2022.2162764.

22. Kim D-Y, Lee J-S, Park S-Y, Kim S-J, Son C-G. Systematic review of randomized controlled trials for chronic fatigue syndrome/myalgic encephalomyelitis (CFS/ME). J Transl Med. 2020;18:1–12.
23. Luedke JC, Vargas G, Jashar DT, Malone LA, Morrow A, Ng R. Neuropsychological functioning of pediatric patients with long COVID. Clin Neuropsychol. 2024;38(8):1855–72. https://doi.org/10.1080/13854046.2024.2344455.
24. Miskowiak K, Pedersen J, Gunnarsson D, Roikjer T, Podlekareva D, Hansen H, Dall C, Johnsen S. Cognitive impairments among patients in a long-COVID clinic: prevalence, pattern and relation to illness severity, work function and quality of life. J Affect Disord. 2023;324:162–9.
25. Moola S, Munn Z, Tufanaru C, Aromataris E, Sears K, Sfetcu R, Currie M, Qureshi R, Mattis P, Lisy K, Mu PF. Chapter 7: Systematic reviews of etiology and risk. In: Joanna Briggs Institute reviewer's manual. The Joanna Briggs Institute; 2017.
26. Mukherjee S, Singer T, Venkatesh A, Choudhury NA, Perez Giraldo GS, Jimenez M, Miller J, Lopez M, Hanson BA, Bawa AP, Batra A, Liotta EM, Koralnik IJ. Vaccination prior to SARS-CoV-2 infection does not affect the neurologic manifestations of long COVID. Brain Commun. 2025;7(1):fcae448. https://doi.org/10.1093/braincomms/fcae448.
27. Oberauer K. Working memory and attention – response to commentaries. J Cogn. 2019;2(1):30. https://doi.org/10.5334/joc.79.
28. Pazukhina E, Andreeva M, Spiridonova E, Bobkova P, Shikhaleva A, El-Taravi Y, Rumyantsev M, Gamirova A, Bairashevskaia A, Petrova P. Prevalence and risk factors of post-COVID-19 condition in adults and children at 6 and 12 months after hospital discharge: a prospective, cohort study in Moscow (StopCOVID). BMC Med. 2022;20(1):244.
29. Pellegrino R, Chiappini E, Licari A, Galli L, Marseglia GL. Prevalence and clinical presentation of long COVID in children: a systematic review. Eur J Pediatr. 2022;181(12):3995–4009.
30. Putri ND, Laksanawati IS, Husada D, Kaswandani N, Prayitno A, Triasih R, Hidayati IS, Asih R, Nurhariansyah R, Cathleen F, Ocviyanti D, Hadinegoro SR, Pelicci D, Bines J, Graham SM. A systematic review of post COVID-19 condition in children and adolescents: gap in evidence from low-and -middle-income countries and the impact of SARS-COV-2 variants. PLoS One. 2025;20(3):e0315815. https://doi.org/10.1371/journal.pone.0315815.
31. Rabiner DL, Carrig MM, Dodge KA. Attention problems and academic achievement: do persistent and earlier-emerging problems have more adverse long-term effects? J Atten Disord. 2016;20(11):946–57. https://doi.org/10.1177/1087054713507974.
32. Roge I, Smane L, Kivite-Urtane A, Pucuka Z, Racko I, Klavina L, Pavare J. Comparison of persistent symptoms after COVID-19 and other non-SARS-CoV-2 infections in children. Front Pediatr. 2021;9:752385.
33. Rucker G, Schwarzer G, Carpenter J. Arcsine test for publication bias in meta-analyses with binary outcomes. Stat Med. 2008;27(5):746–63. https://doi.org/10.1002/sim.2971.
34. Sanal-Hayes NEM, McLaughlin M, Hayes LD, Mair JL, Ormerod J, Carless D, Hilliard N, Meach R, Ingram J, Sculthorpe NF. A scoping review of 'Pacing' for management of Myalgic Encephalomyelitis/Chronic Fatigue Syndrome (ME/CFS): lessons learned for the long COVID pandemic. J Transl Med. 2023;21(1):720. https://doi.org/10.1186/s12967-023-04587-5.
35. Scarselli V, Calderoni D, Terrinoni A, Davico C, Pruccoli G, Denina M, Carducci C, Smarrazzo A, Martucci M, Presicce M, Marcotulli D, Arletti L, Ferrara M, Garazzino S, Mariani R, Campana A, Vitiello B. A neuropsychiatric assessment of children with previous SARS-CoV-2 infection. J Clin Med. 2023;12(12) https://doi.org/10.3390/jcm12123917.
36. Siegel ALM, Castel AD. The role of attention in remembering important item-location associations. Mem Cognit. 2018;46(8):1248–62. https://doi.org/10.3758/s13421-018-0834-4.
37. Sterky E, Olsson-Åkefeldt S, Hertting O, Herlenius E, Alfven T, Rinder MR, Rhedin S, Hildenwall H. Persistent symptoms in Swedish children after hospitalisation due to COVID-19. Acta Paediatrica (Oslo, Norway: 1992). 2021;110(9):2578.
38. The Jamovi Project. Jamovi (Version 2.4) [Computer Software]. 2024. Retreived from https://jamovi.org

39. Veritas Health Innovation. Covidence systematic review software. 2024.
40. Zheng Y-B, Zeng N, Yuan K, Tian S-S, Yang Y-B, Gao N, Chen X, Zhang A-Y, Kondratiuk AL, Shi P-P. Prevalence and risk factor for long COVID in children and adolescents: a meta-analysis and systematic review. J Infect Public Health. 2023;16(5):660–72.

Long Covid or Post-Covid -19 Neurological Syndrome?

12

Tissa Wijeratne and Sheila Crewther

12.1 Introduction

The global discourse surrounding long-term consequences of COVID has been shaped primarily by the term Long COVID. While this term has served a useful purpose in elevating public awareness and acknowledging the chronic effects of SARS-CoV-2 infection, it has also contributed to conceptual ambiguity. The term Long COVID has come to represent a diverse constellation of symptoms ranging from fatigue and breathlessness to joint pain, chest tightness, anxiety, and brain fog. In doing so, it risks obscuring the specific biological and clinical patterns that define distinct syndromes within the broader post-COVID condition.

One such syndrome is Post-COVID Neurological Syndrome, or PCNS. This condition is increasingly recognized in peer-reviewed literature and clinical settings as a cluster of neurological symptoms with consistent features. These include persistent cognitive impairment, slowed thinking, poor concentration, altered sensory perception, autonomic instability, and disturbances in mood and sleep. For many patients, these symptoms began soon after the acute infection and have persisted for months or even years, often in the absence of any structural damage detectable through conventional imaging.

As new cohorts of affected individuals continue to emerge, there is growing concern that the lack of precise classification is delaying diagnosis, hindering research, and limiting access to care. Without a clear distinction between PCNS and other non-neurological manifestations of Long COVID, clinical pathways remain

T. Wijeratne (✉)
Department of Neurology and Stroke, La Trobe University, St. Albans, VIC, Australia
e-mail: tissa.wijeratne@wh.org.au

S. Crewther
Western Health, La Trobe University, Melbourne, VIC, Australia
e-mail: S.Crewther@latrobe.edu.au

T. Wijeratne, S. Crewther (eds.), *Post Covid-19 Neurological Syndrome*,
https://doi.org/10.1007/978-3-032-14995-4_12

fragmented. Patients with primarily neurological symptoms are often referred between specialists, subjected to unnecessary investigations, or told their symptoms are psychological in origin. Clinicians on the front lines are left to manage these patients with minimal guidance, few evidence based tools, and no targeted treatment protocols. The result is not only clinical inefficiency but also profound patient frustration and distress.

In this chapter, we propose that the term Long COVID, while valuable in early phases of the pandemic, is now insufficient to address the complexity of post-infectious outcomes. The time has come to delineate PCNS as a specific diagnostic category with its own research and care agenda. This distinction is not just semantic. It carries real implications for clinical management, policy development, disability support, and research funding allocation. It also honors the lived experience of patients, many of whom have reported cognitive decline, loss of function, and mental fatigue that interfere with daily life in deeply disabling ways.

The distinction between PCNS and Long COVID also reflects a more accurate understanding of disease mechanisms. Research is beginning to reveal specific immune and inflammatory pathways that may drive ongoing neurological dysfunction following COVID. These include microglial activation, persistent cytokine elevation, disruption to the blood brain barrier, and impaired cerebral perfusion. Importantly, these findings suggest that PCNS is not simply a stress response or a vague post-viral syndrome. It is a biologically grounded disorder that affects key systems in the brain and nervous system. Ongoing studies using neuroimaging, blood biomarkers, and neuropsychological assessment are helping to build a more detailed picture of the mechanisms underlying PCNS and their potential therapeutic targets.

Another reason to separate PCNS from the wider Long COVID framework is the unique trajectory of recovery. While many individuals with Long COVID experience multisystem symptoms that gradually improve with time, those with PCNS may follow a more protracted and relapsing course. Some patients report brief periods of improvement followed by sudden cognitive crashes. Others experience gradual worsening of brain function despite stable respiratory or cardiovascular parameters. This mismatch between physical recovery and cognitive wellbeing underscores the need for specialized follow up and dedicated rehabilitation pathways. A generalist model of Long COVID care, while valuable in early screening, cannot replace the need for neurological expertise and systems based diagnostic frameworks.

The argument for defining PCNS as a distinct syndrome has also been supported by global health bodies and national policy initiatives. The World Health Organization now acknowledges neurological post-COVID symptoms as a major domain of concern, and calls for research to better understand their nature and impact. In 2023, the Australian Parliament released its inquiry into Long COVID and repeated COVID infections. The report emphasized the need for investment in multidisciplinary care, education for health professionals, and research funding to explore the biological basis of persistent post-viral symptoms, including those affecting brain function. These developments signal a policy shift toward more refined classification and targeted responses to the long term consequences of COVID.

It is important to recognize that many patients still identify strongly with the term Long COVID. It has provided a sense of community, advocacy, and validation when few formal structures existed to support them. Any proposal to define PCNS separately must not undermine the efforts or identity of Long COVID advocates. Instead, it should be seen as an evolution in our understanding, one that allows for better care, stronger science, and a more accurate public health response. Much as the understanding of autoimmune diseases expanded from broad categories into more precise subtypes, so too must our framing of post-COVID conditions.

This chapter aims to present a clear rationale for recognizing PCNS as its own clinical entity. We will examine the symptom clusters, patient trajectories, and emerging biological evidence that distinguish it from other forms of Long COVID. We will explore the risks of continued diagnostic ambiguity and the benefits of clinical precision. We will also consider how new models of care—including systems neuroscience tools, longitudinal monitoring, and explainable artificial intelligence—can support this refined approach. Finally, we will reflect on the ethical and communication challenges that come with renaming and reframing syndromes in real time.

In short, this chapter is not a rejection of Long COVID. Rather, it is an invitation to deepen our understanding and respond to what the science and patients are clearly telling us. PCNS is real, disabling, and biologically distinct. It deserves recognition, research, and resources. Defining it clearly is the first step in delivering the support that patients and clinicians urgently need.

12.2 Framing the Clinical Case for PCNS

The rapid growth of clinical cases following COVID has exposed a critical gap in our understanding of long-term neurological complications. Among the most widely reported symptoms is brain fog, which encompasses poor concentration, slowed thinking, memory lapses, and general cognitive fatigue. This symptom alone has disrupted the lives of thousands, preventing return to work, limiting independence, and deeply affecting quality of life. Although originally lumped under the broader term Long COVID, there is now compelling evidence that a distinct neurological syndrome exists—Post-COVID Neurological Syndrome, or PCNS.

From a clinical perspective, PCNS presents in a consistent and recognizable pattern. It often emerges within weeks of a COVID infection, persists beyond the expected recovery period, and follows a trajectory that does not necessarily correlate with the severity of the initial illness. Many affected individuals were never hospitalized or even considered high risk during their acute COVID episode, yet they now face persistent brain-related symptoms that resemble those seen in acquired brain injury, post-viral encephalopathy, and other neurological disorders. This disconnect challenges traditional models of symptom progression and demands new diagnostic thinking.

What makes PCNS more than a collection of symptoms is the way it manifests across key domains of nervous system function. Cognitive impairments are often accompanied by sleep disturbances, sensory sensitivity, dysautonomia, mood changes, and post-exertional symptom worsening. This constellation points to a multi-level disruption of brain and systemic regulation, consistent with conditions involving neuroinflammation, disrupted neurovascular function, and altered homeostasis.

Clinicians have described a frustrating cycle of care. Patients with PCNS symptoms are referred from general practitioners to neurologists, from neurologists to psychiatrists, and from psychiatrists back to primary care. Standard imaging is often normal. Routine blood tests may show no abnormalities. With no clear diagnosis, many are told their symptoms are anxiety-related or psychosomatic. This not only delays care, but also contributes to stigma and undermines patient trust.

A well-defined clinical case for PCNS would offer clarity, streamline care, and accelerate research. It would enable clinicians to use a structured approach to evaluate symptoms, apply consistent diagnostic criteria, and rule in PCNS rather than only ruling out other disorders. It would support development of symptom severity scales and facilitate rehabilitation planning. Just as multiple sclerosis and Parkinson's disease transitioned from loosely defined syndromes to clearly categorized neurological disorders, PCNS must now take that step.

Defining PCNS also allows for differentiation from other aspects of Long COVID. Not all people with Long COVID experience significant cognitive issues. Likewise, not all individuals with PCNS have respiratory or cardiac symptoms. Recognizing the unique clinical footprint of PCNS enables care to be tailored more effectively and allows multidisciplinary teams to work from a shared understanding.

The clinical case for PCNS is not just a matter of naming. It is a foundation for improving outcomes, informing patients, designing trials, and educating providers. It moves us from confusion to clarity, from fragmented care to integrated pathways, and from disbelief to recognition. For the sake of the millions affected worldwide, this transition is both overdue and essential.

12.3 Data Driven Arguments and Emerging Biological Evidence

Scientific evidence continues to build in support of PCNS as a biologically grounded neurological disorder rather than a psychological or functional condition. Recent studies have revealed measurable changes in brain structure, persistent markers of immune dysregulation, and patterns of neuroinflammation in people experiencing post-COVID brain fog and cognitive impairment. These findings lend strong credibility to the argument that PCNS should be treated as a distinct neurological condition.

Recent advances in sensory neuroimmunology have opened a compelling new frontier in our understanding of Post-COVID Neurological Syndrome [21]. The classic division between immune surveillance and neural sensation is rapidly dissolving. A growing body of evidence now reveals that sensory neurons are not passive conduits of external stimuli, but active participants in immune signaling, inflammation regulation, and tissue homeostasis. This convergence of immunology and neurobiology adds critical depth to how we conceptualize persistent neurological symptoms in PCNS.

As outlined by Kim and Artis in their landmark 2025 perspective, both the immune and nervous systems share foundational capabilities: sensing, responding, and adapting to internal and external threats [21]. Sensory neurons, particularly those in the dorsal root ganglia, have been shown to respond directly to inflammatory cytokines such as interleukin 6 and tumor necrosis factor alpha. These cytokines can enhance pain, fatigue, and itch not only through peripheral inflammation but also by activating neurogenic pathways that sustain and amplify symptom burdens over time. The implication is profound: inflammation in PCNS may not just affect neurons—it may be co-constructed with them through a bidirectional neuro-immune dialogue.

Importantly, this interface is not limited to pain perception. Cytokines such as IL-31 and IL-33 have been found to engage directly with somatosensory neurons, evoking itch and hypersensitivity through mechanisms remarkably similar to neurotransmission. These insights have led to the development of successful biologic treatments for chronic inflammatory conditions such as atopic dermatitis. If these cytokines are also dysregulated in PCNS—as preliminary studies suggest—then targeting their neural receptors may hold therapeutic promise for treating persistent symptoms such as brain fog, sensory sensitivity, and autonomic imbalance.

The interaction between environmental cues and sensory neurons is another critical axis in PCNS biology. Microbial toxins, allergens, and metabolic products are increasingly recognized for their ability to modulate neuroimmune circuits. In the gut, respiratory tract, and skin, sensory neurons detect bacterial components and communicate danger signals to local immune cells. In the context of PCNS, it is plausible that a similar system is activated or dysregulated following COVID infection, particularly in individuals with predisposing immune profiles or altered microbiota. This may help explain the variable symptom expression, chronicity, and flare-like nature of PCNS.

A central mediator of these interactions is the neuropeptide CGRP (calcitonin gene-related peptide), which can promote or suppress inflammation depending on the local tissue environment. For example, CGRP has been shown to impair antiviral immunity in cancer models while supporting wound healing and immune tolerance in mucosal surfaces. In PCNS, altered CGRP signaling could contribute to both the persistence of symptoms and the variability in immune resolution, especially if sensory neurons are chronically activated or structurally altered after viral exposure.

These discoveries support the view that PCNS is not a purely downstream consequence of immune activation or vascular injury. Rather, it may be rooted in a complex and dynamic interplay between peripheral neurons and immune cells. Understanding this interplay requires a systems neuroscience approach, one that does not isolate organ systems but instead investigates how networks of signaling, sensing, and regulation influence recovery or deterioration.

Taken together, the sensory neuroimmune frontier offers a rich and largely untapped framework for explaining the sustained neurological dysfunction observed in PCNS. Future research should explore how specific cytokine-receptor interactions, neuropeptide signaling, and microbiota-derived cues modulate this interface in affected individuals. This will not only clarify pathogenesis but also inform therapeutic development with the potential to interrupt chronic symptom loops at their source.

Further advancing the biological basis of Post-COVID Neurological Syndrome, Janket and colleagues propose a compelling mechanism rooted in neuroimmune signaling [20]. They emphasize the central role of substance P, a well-studied tachykinin neuropeptide, in linking the immune and nervous systems. Substance P is expressed throughout the body and actively participates in a wide range of physiological and pathological processes. These include inflammation, pain perception, gastrointestinal regulation, respiratory control, and modulation of immune responses. What makes substance P particularly relevant to PCNS is its role in bidirectional communication between immune cells and neurons. Immune cells located near nerve endings can release cytokines and other factors that trigger or modulate neuronal activity. Conversely, sensory neurons can release substance P to amplify immune signaling. This creates a self-reinforcing cycle that may help explain the persistent, fluctuating symptoms seen in individuals with PCNS.

The authors propose that this neuroimmune crosstalk may serve as a foundational driver of the diverse symptoms associated with long COVID, including brain fog, headaches, fatigue, gastrointestinal disturbances, and autonomic dysfunction. This insight aligns with clinical observations that PCNS symptoms often involve overlapping systems, particularly the brain-gut axis and autonomic control loops. Substance P is known to be a key modulator in both. Its dysregulation could therefore produce widespread downstream effects, from cognitive slowing and mood changes to irritable bowel patterns and altered heart rate variability. This unified model offers a possible biological explanation for how a single triggering event—SARS-CoV-2 infection—could give rise to such a wide range of persistent and seemingly unrelated symptoms.

Importantly, the review highlights a therapeutic opportunity. If substance P and its receptors play a central role in sustaining PCNS, then targeting this pathway could offer a new approach to treatment. Several neurokinin receptor antagonists have already been developed for other inflammatory and pain-related conditions. These could be repurposed or refined for use in post-viral syndromes. While clinical trials will be necessary, the mechanistic clarity offered by this model provides a strong rationale for pursuing such interventions. It also offers clinicians and researchers a valuable framework for integrating disparate PCNS symptoms under a single biological narrative.

The findings further underscore the need for a systems biology approach to PCNS. It is not sufficient to study inflammation, neuronal injury, or immune dysregulation in isolation. Rather, these elements interact within dynamic networks that may be mediated by neuropeptides such as substance P. Mapping these interactions with greater precision—across time and across patient populations—will be essential for designing better diagnostic tools and personalized treatment strategies. As Janket and colleagues make clear, we are only beginning to understand the complexity of post-viral neuroimmune syndromes, yet by studying molecules like substance P, we gain a foothold into a much broader landscape of neuroinflammation and repair.

One important reason to revisit the biology we understood well before the pandemic is highlighted in a 2016 study by Schlereth and colleagues [24]. Their research demonstrated the complex interplay between the neuropeptides substance P and calcitonin gene-related peptide (CGRP), both of which are released from sensory nerve endings and known to influence pain, inflammation, and vascular responses. The study showed that while substance P caused transient vasodilation and plasma extravasation in the skin, co-administration of CGRP altered these responses significantly, attenuating the early vasodilatory effect while amplifying the inflammatory leakage. This nuanced interaction provides a vivid example of how small molecular signals can create diverse and sometimes opposing effects depending on concentration, timing, and tissue context. These findings remind us that many of the mechanisms likely at play in PCNS were already known in other domains of neurology and immunology. We now have a responsibility to integrate this foundational knowledge into our post-COVID clinical thinking and bring it back to the bedside to better understand and treat complex, multi-systemic symptoms such as brain fog and dysautonomia.

A recent study by Gao and Bayraktutan adds powerful support to the argument that PCNS shares underlying biology with other complex brain disorders such as migraine and possibly neurodegenerative diseases [4]. Their work shows that substance P, a neuropeptide already implicated in pain and inflammation, can cause a reversible breakdown of the blood brain barrier. This disruption happens without changing the levels of tight junction proteins, which were once believed to be the key drivers of barrier integrity. Instead, substance P acts through cellular stress mechanisms involving the RhoA and ROCK signaling pathways, weakening the brain's protective shield in a time-dependent manner. This discovery is highly relevant for PCNS, where fluctuating symptoms like brain fog, cognitive crashes, and sensory hypersensitivities may be linked to subtle and recurring disturbances in blood brain barrier function. Notably, migraine research has also implicated substance P and CGRP in barrier disruption and neurogenic inflammation. By recognizing this shared biology, we are better positioned to move away from symptom silos and begin thinking about PCNS as part of a broader category of neuroimmune interface disorders. It is time we apply what we know from migraine and pain research to the daily care and science of PCNS [29–31].

The renewed scientific focus on substance P in migraine research reinforces its importance in neuroimmune biology. As highlighted by Pellesi and Edvinsson, earlier therapeutic strategies targeting substance P were set aside after disappointing results [23]. However, the recent success of peptide-targeted treatments for CGRP and PACAP has reignited interest in substance P as a critical mediator of migraine and other neurological disorders. This shift in thinking aligns closely with what we observe in PCNS, where fluctuating symptoms, neurovascular instability, and inflammatory cascades suggest a shared pathway. Revisiting substance P with modern tools and trial designs is not just a chance to improve migraine care but an opportunity to apply that same insight to post-viral neuroimmune syndromes like PCNS. It is time to bring these threads together.

Imaging studies using functional MRI have demonstrated altered connectivity in key brain networks, especially those involved in memory, attention, and executive function. In some individuals, these changes resemble patterns seen in other neuroinflammatory disorders such as multiple sclerosis or post-encephalitic syndromes. Reports have also noted reduced grey matter volume and abnormalities in white matter microstructure in patients who continue to experience symptoms several months after their COVID infection.

Blood based biomarker studies further support the biological distinctiveness of PCNS. Elevated levels of cytokines such as interleukin 6, interleukin 1 beta, and tumor necrosis factor alpha have been found in PCNS cohorts, pointing toward a pro-inflammatory state. Other studies have identified signs of disrupted blood brain barrier integrity, increased microglial activation, and elevated markers of oxidative stress. These processes can impair synaptic transmission, reduce neurogenesis, and disrupt communication between brain regions—all of which are consistent with the clinical symptoms observed.

Electrophysiological and neuropsychological testing also reveals consistent abnormalities. Patients with PCNS often show reduced processing speed, impaired working memory, and difficulty with sustained attention. These deficits are quantifiable and reproducible, offering objective correlates to subjective complaints of brain fog and mental fatigue. They also provide potential endpoints for clinical trials.

Emerging evidence also points to metabolic and autonomic dysfunction as important contributors. Individuals with PCNS may exhibit altered cortisol rhythms, mitochondrial stress, or impaired autonomic regulation. These dysfunctions may not always be visible on conventional tests but can significantly impact cognition, energy levels, and emotional resilience. This reinforces the need for a systems level approach to diagnosis and management.

Importantly, these biological patterns are found even in individuals who had mild or asymptomatic COVID infections [19, 22, 26–28]. This disproves the notion that PCNS is a post-intensive care phenomenon or solely the result of psychological trauma. It also explains why so many people have developed disabling symptoms despite having no prior health concerns and no complications during their acute infection.

Together, these findings challenge the outdated view that post-viral syndromes are too vague to be treated seriously. Instead, they show that PCNS is biologically real, measurable, and deserving of dedicated scientific inquiry. Ongoing longitudinal cohort studies, brain bank initiatives, and international collaborations will help refine our understanding and point the way to biomarker informed therapies.

For PCNS to be properly addressed, the science must continue to evolve and be integrated into routine care. This means investing in data collection tools, harmonizing diagnostic criteria, and supporting interdisciplinary teams that combine neurology, immunology, psychiatry, and rehabilitation medicine. It also means acknowledging that the current evidence base, though incomplete, is already strong enough to justify recognition of PCNS as a distinct and serious condition that warrants urgent attention

12.4 Implications for Care, Research, and Health Policy

Recognizing PCNS as a distinct condition has far-reaching implications for healthcare delivery, clinical research, and public health policy. First and foremost, it allows for the development of specific care pathways that reflect the unique needs of individuals with post-COVID neurological symptoms. Without a formal diagnostic category, patients with PCNS are often excluded from appropriate services, fall between specialties, and face inconsistent standards of care. Designating PCNS as a recognized neurological disorder will facilitate the creation of dedicated clinics, improve access to multidisciplinary rehabilitation, and promote standardization of treatment approaches.

From a care perspective, the integration of PCNS into clinical practice requires new models built around collaboration. Neurologists, immunologists, psychiatrists, physiotherapists, occupational therapists, speech pathologists, and general practitioners must work together in a coordinated manner. No single specialist holds the entire picture of PCNS, and siloed care risks delaying diagnosis and fragmenting treatment. Multidisciplinary teams should be supported by clear referral pathways, diagnostic checklists, and continuing education that reflects the evolving science of PCNS.

The implications for rehabilitation are especially significant. Many individuals with PCNS report post-exertional symptom exacerbation, fluctuating fatigue, cognitive crashes, and autonomic instability. Traditional rehabilitation protocols may not be appropriate for this patient population. Instead, care plans must emphasize pacing, cognitive rest, symptom tracking, and gradual reintroduction of activity based on individual tolerance. Tailored interventions informed by neuropsychological profiling and patient reported outcomes will be essential to avoid harm and promote sustainable recovery.

In terms of research, formally defining PCNS opens the door to targeted investigations. It allows for more precise cohort selection, consistent outcome measurement, and reliable identification of disease subtypes. This will accelerate the development of diagnostic tools, therapeutic strategies, and personalized rehabilitation models. Current research efforts remain fragmented and underfunded, with limited coordination across centers and countries. A unified research agenda, supported by large-scale longitudinal studies and collaborative networks, is urgently needed.

Biobanking, real-world data integration, and digital health monitoring will be critical components of this agenda. By collecting standardized biological samples and linking them with cognitive assessments, neuroimaging, and wearable data, researchers can identify biomarkers that predict onset, severity, and recovery trajectories. This kind of systems-based research will also support the development of explainable artificial intelligence models that assist in diagnosis, triage, and treatment personalization.

At the policy level, the case for recognizing PCNS carries implications for funding, service design, and workforce training. Health systems must allocate resources for the establishment of PCNS-focused clinics, mobile health units, and telehealth services. Insurance schemes and disability frameworks must be updated to accommodate the reality of post-COVID neurological impairment, particularly among working-age adults who have lost employment or functional independence. Governments and professional bodies must invest in workforce development to ensure that clinicians are trained to recognize and manage PCNS appropriately.

Public health messaging also plays a crucial role. Clear communication that PCNS is real, common, and treatable can help reduce stigma and encourage people to seek care. It can also reinforce the importance of COVID prevention strategies such as vaccination, given the potential for long term neurological effects even after mild infections. Educational campaigns should be co-designed with people who have lived experience of PCNS to ensure they are relatable, accurate, and impactful.

Importantly, the social and economic cost of inaction is high. Lost productivity, increased healthcare utilization, long-term disability, and psychological distress all add to the burden of PCNS on individuals, families, and society. Investing in research, services, and early intervention is not only a moral imperative—it is economically sound policy.

Global collaboration will be essential. As PCNS transcends borders, it presents an opportunity for international cooperation in data sharing, trial coordination, and health system innovation. Multilateral organizations like the World Health Organization can play a convening role, bringing together countries to align research priorities, standardize diagnostic criteria, and ensure equitable access to care. Low and middle income countries must be supported in building capacity to detect and manage PCNS, to avoid deepening global health inequities [1–3, 5–18].

Lastly, patients and caregivers must be recognized as co-creators of the future of PCNS care. Their insights into symptom patterns, daily challenges, and treatment experiences are essential for shaping responsive health systems. Patient advocacy groups have already led much of the progress in raising awareness and demanding recognition for Long COVID and PCNS. Their continued leadership will be vital as we build a more inclusive, evidence-based, and humane approach to post-COVID neurological care.

In conclusion, recognizing PCNS as a distinct condition is not just a matter of science. It is a turning point for brain health globally. PCNS is a common and disabling condition driven by chronic, low grade neuroinflammation affecting key circuits in the brain. It is not rare or mysterious. It is real, measurable, and deeply disruptive to daily life. Failing to act now risks prolonging suffering and deepening inequality.

We must respond with urgency and clarity. Academic centres, clinicians, patients, and carers need to work together to investigate this condition properly and create meaningful solutions. We already have many of the tools we need. What we need now is coordinated action. We must bring the biology we have long understood, about neuropeptides, immune signalling, and barrier integrity, back to the clinical frontline.

This work directly aligns with global initiatives such as World Brain Day and the WHO's Intersectoral Global Action Plan. These frameworks call for multisectoral cooperation and real investment in neurological care. PCNS is a test case. If we succeed here, we build the future of precision neurology and person-centred recovery. With smart research, shared data, and the lived knowledge of those affected, we can change the course of this condition starting today.

This is exactly what we have been hearing from thousands of PCNS patients and families we have been meeting and caring for in Melbourne, Australia since our original description of the condition in 2020 [25]. Their experiences have shaped our understanding and deepened our commitment to this field. These are people living with daily challenges who are asking for recognition, care, and hope. It is time to answer that call with unified purpose and determined action.

References

1. Amatya S, Khan E, Kagzi Y, Akkus S, Gupta R, Hansen N, Wen S, Jaiswal S, Sriwastava S. Disease characteristics of NMOSD and their relationship with disease burden: observations from a large single-center cohort. J Neurol Sci. 2024;467:123311.
2. Avan A, Digaleh H, Di Napoli M, Stranges S, Behrouz R, Shojaeianbabaei G, Amiri A, Tabrizi R, Mokhber N, Spence JD, Azarpazhooh MR. Socioeconomic status and stroke incidence, prevalence, mortality, and worldwide burden: an ecological analysis from the Global Burden of Disease Study 2017. BMC Med. 2019;17:191.
3. Azarpazhooh MR, Morovatdar N, Avan A, Phan TG, Divani AA, Yassi N, Stranges S, Silver B, Biller J, Tokazebani Belasi M, Kazemi Neya S, Khorram B, Frydman A, Nilanont Y, Onorati E, Di Napoli M. COVID-19 pandemic and burden of non-communicable diseases: an ecological study on data of 185 countries. J Stroke Cerebrovasc Dis. 2020;29:105089.
4. Gao X, Bayraktutan U. Substance P reversibly compromises the integrity and function of blood-brain barrier. Peptides. 2023;167:171048.
5. Global, regional, and national burden of neurological disorders during 1990–2015: a systematic analysis for the Global Burden of Disease Study 2015. Lancet Neurol. 2017;16:877–97.
6. Global, regional, and national burden of meningitis, 1990–2016: a systematic analysis for the Global Burden of Disease Study 2016. Lancet Neurol. 2018a;17:1061–82.
7. Global, regional, and national burden of motor neuron diseases 1990–2016: a systematic analysis for the Global Burden of Disease Study 2016. Lancet Neurol. 2018b;17:1083–97.
8. Global, regional, and national burden of brain and other CNS cancer, 1990–2016: a systematic analysis for the Global Burden of Disease Study 2016. Lancet Neurol. 2019a;18:376–93.
9. Global, regional, and national burden of epilepsy, 1990–2016: a systematic analysis for the Global Burden of Disease Study 2016. Lancet Neurol. 2019b;18:357–75.
10. Global, regional, and national burden of stroke and its risk factors, 1990–2019: a systematic analysis for the Global Burden of Disease Study 2019. Lancet Neurol. 2021;20:795–820.
11. Global burden of chronic respiratory diseases and risk factors, 1990–2019: an update from the Global Burden of Disease Study 2019. EClinicalMedicine. 2023;59:101936.
12. Global age-sex-specific mortality, life expectancy, and population estimates in 204 countries and territories and 811 subnational locations, 1950–2021, and the impact of the COVID-19 pandemic: a comprehensive demographic analysis for the Global Burden of Disease Study 2021. Lancet. 2024a;403:1989–2056.

13. Global burden of 288 causes of death and life expectancy decomposition in 204 countries and territories and 811 subnational locations, 1990–2021: a systematic analysis for the Global Burden of Disease Study 2021. Lancet. 2024b;403:2100–132.
14. Global fertility in 204 countries and territories, 1950–2021, with forecasts to 2100: a comprehensive demographic analysis for the Global Burden of Disease Study 2021. Lancet. 2024c;403:2057–99.
15. Global, regional, and national burden of urolithiasis in 204 countries and territories, 2000–2021: a systematic analysis for the Global Burden of Disease Study 2021. EClinicalMedicine. 2024d;78:102924.
16. Global, regional, and national burden of epilepsy, 1990–2021: a systematic analysis for the Global Burden of Disease Study 2021. Lancet Public Health. 2025a;10:e203–227.
17. Global, regional, and national prevalence of child and adolescent overweight and obesity, 1990–2021, with forecasts to 2050: a forecasting study for the Global Burden of Disease Study 2021. Lancet. 2025b;405:785–812.
18. Global, regional, and national progress towards the 2030 global nutrition targets and forecasts to 2050: a systematic analysis for the Global Burden of Disease Study 2021. Lancet. 2025c;404:2543–83.
19. Hassan EB, Phu S, Warburton E, Humaith N, Wijeratne T. Frailty in stroke – a narrated review. Life (Basel). 2021:11.
20. Janket SJ, Fraser DD, Baird AE, Tamimi F, Sohaei D, Conte HA, Prassas I, Diamandis EP. Tachykinins and the potential causal factors for post-COVID-19 condition. Lancet Microbe. 2023;4:e642–50.
21. Kim BS, Artis D. The sensory neuroimmune frontier. Immunity. 2025;58:1033–9.
22. Ma Y, Deng J, Liu Q, Du M, Liu M, Liu J. Long-term consequences of asymptomatic SARS-CoV-2 infection: a systematic review and meta-analysis. Int J Environ Res Public Health. 2023;20.
23. Pellesi L, Edvinsson L. Revisiting substance P in migraine: a methodological approach inspired by anti-CGRP and anti-PACAP success. J Headache Pain. 2025;26:22.
24. Schlereth T, Schukraft J, Krämer-Best HH, Geber C, Ackermann T, Birklein F. Interaction of calcitonin gene related peptide (CGRP) and substance P (SP) in human skin. Neuropeptides. 2016;59:57–62.
25. Wijeratne T, Crewther S. Post-COVID 19 Neurological Syndrome (PCNS); a novel syndrome with challenges for the global neurology community. J Neurol Sci. 2020;419:117179.
26. Wijeratne T, Crewther SG. A systems neuroscience approach to diagnosis and rehabilitation of post COVID neurological syndrome based on the Systems Neuroscience Test Battery (SNTB) Study Protocol. NeuroRehabilitation. 2025;56:37–47.
27. Wijeratne T, Wijeratne C. Clinical utility of serial systemic immune inflammation indices (SSIIi) in the context of post covid-19 neurological syndrome (PCNS). J Neurol Sci. 2021;423:117356.
28. Wijeratne T, Gillard Crewther S, Sales C, Karimi L. COVID-19 pathophysiology predicts that ischemic stroke occurrence is an expectation, not an exception – a systematic review. Front Neurol. 2020;11:607221.
29. Wijeratne T, Sales C, Wijeratne C, Karimi L, Jakovljevic M. Systematic review of existing stroke guidelines: case for a change. Biomed Res Int. 2022;2022:5514793.
30. Wijeratne T, Murphy MJ, Wijeratne C, Martelletti P, Karimi L, Apostolopoulos V, Sales C, Riddell N, Crewther SG. Serial systemic immune inflammation indices: markers of acute migraine events or indicators of persistent inflammatory status? J Headache Pain. 2025a;26:7.
31. Wijeratne T, Murphy MJ, Wijeratne C, Martelletti P, Karimi L, Apostolopoulos V, Sales C, Riddell N, Crewther SG. Serial systemic immune inflammation indices: markers of acute migraine events or indicators of persistent inflammatory status? J Headache Pain. 2025b;26:7.

13 Post-COVID Neurological Syndrome: A Turning Point for Brain Health and Sustainable Development

Tissa Wijeratne and Sheila Crewther

13.1 Introduction

The global COVID 19 pandemic has challenged every dimension of modern healthcare, revealing the fragility of systems and the far reaching effects of viral illness beyond the acute infection phase. As the world transitions into the post-pandemic era, there is growing recognition of a persistent and often debilitating condition that continues to affect millions long after their initial recovery from SARS CoV 2 infection. This condition, now recognized by increasing numbers of clinicians and researchers, is Post-COVID Neurological Syndrome (PCNS).

PCNS refers to a constellation of neurological, cognitive, autonomic, and psychiatric symptoms that persist or emerge following acute COVID 19. These symptoms often include cognitive impairment ("brain fog"), chronic fatigue, mood disturbances, sleep dysregulation, dysautonomia, sensory changes, and headache. Unlike the acute viral illness which typically follows a predictable course, PCNS is insidious, lingering, and for many patients, disabling. It disrupts personal, social, and occupational functioning and contributes significantly to the global burden of disease.

Since the initial reports in early 2020, PCNS has become a prominent example of a post-infectious syndrome that bridges neurology, immunology, psychiatry, and rehabilitation medicine. Despite this, it remains poorly understood, inconsistently defined, and grossly under recognized in clinical settings. The persistence of diagnostic uncertainty has not only hindered effective management but also led to

T. Wijeratne (✉)
Department of Neurology and Stroke, La Trobe University, St. Albans, VIC, Australia
e-mail: tissa.wijeratne@wh.org.au

S. Crewther
Western Health, La Trobe University, Melbourne, VIC, Australia
e-mail: S.Crewther@latrobe.edu.au

T. Wijeratne, S. Crewther (eds.), *Post Covid-19 Neurological Syndrome*,
https://doi.org/10.1007/978-3-032-14995-4_13

widespread dismissal of patients' experiences, thereby deepening stigma and delaying appropriate intervention.

The need to define PCNS as a distinct clinical entity is no longer a matter of academic debate. Rather, it is a public health imperative. PCNS is common, real, and measurable. Emerging evidence strongly supports the role of chronic low grade neuroinflammation, immune dysregulation, microvascular injury, and impaired blood brain barrier function as core mechanisms underpinning this syndrome. Importantly, these mechanisms are not new. They draw upon decades of knowledge from neuroimmunology, headache medicine, and post-viral encephalopathies. What is new is the scale of the problem and the opportunity to act with urgency, purpose, and innovation.

The World Health Organization has recognized the enduring impact of neurological disorders through its Intersectoral Global Action Plan (IGAP) on epilepsy and other neurological conditions. This landmark strategy calls for the inclusion of brain health across all stages of life, better surveillance, more equitable care, and cross disciplinary collaboration. PCNS exemplifies each of these needs. It is a condition that affects people across the lifespan, with a disproportionate burden among women, frontline workers, those with pre-existing vulnerabilities, and populations in low and middle income countries.

In our own clinical experience, spanning from the earliest days of the pandemic, we have encountered thousands of individuals in Melbourne presenting with persistent post-COVID symptoms affecting their cognitive and neurological function. These patients are not isolated cases. They represent a growing and under supported patient population. Their symptoms are frequently dismissed, under investigated, and left to be managed in silos. Many find themselves caught between multiple medical specialties, none of which fully recognize or take ownership of their condition.

The invisibility of PCNS is made worse by the absence of structural diagnostic codes, targeted funding, and care pathways. Unlike stroke or epilepsy, PCNS lacks the institutional infrastructure that typically guides research, treatment development, and healthcare delivery. This absence has created a vacuum, one that patients are often left to navigate on their own. The result is lost productivity, deteriorating quality of life, increased healthcare use, and significant psychological distress.

There is an urgent need to address this crisis through a systems based lens. PCNS is not a simple post-viral fatigue. It is a multisystem brain disorder driven by ongoing neuroimmune activity. It requires the same level of attention, investment, and coordinated response as other neurological conditions. Research must focus not only on pathophysiology, but also on diagnostics, biomarkers, imaging, cognitive assessment, rehabilitation, and patient reported outcomes. These domains must be integrated into national research strategies and aligned with international efforts under WHO and World Federation of Neurology frameworks.

Equally important is the inclusion of lived experience in shaping the research and policy agenda. The voices of patients and carers have been instrumental in bringing PCNS to the attention of the medical and scientific community. Their advocacy has helped reframe what was once dismissed as anxiety or deconditioning into a serious, biologically based neurological syndrome. Moving forward, patient centered research must become the standard, not the exception.

The Sustainable Development Goals, particularly SDG 3 which promotes health and wellbeing for all at all ages, offer a powerful framework for responding to PCNS. Failure to act risks widening the health equity gap, particularly in communities already facing barriers to neurological care. PCNS is not just a medical issue, it is a social justice issue. Women, migrants, Indigenous populations, people with disabilities, and workers in precarious employment are more likely to suffer from PCNS and less likely to receive appropriate care.

The economic consequences are no less serious. PCNS contributes to loss of income, increased disability claims, early retirement, and rising demand for healthcare services. In high income countries, the impact on workforce participation is beginning to be felt. In lower income settings, the consequences are more severe, where absence of access to rehabilitation services, digital health tools, and interdisciplinary care leaves entire populations at risk of being forgotten.

Technology has an important role to play in reshaping the PCNS landscape. Mobile health platforms, artificial intelligence driven tools, remote cognitive assessment, and telemedicine offer scalable and low cost solutions for both diagnosis and monitoring. These innovations can help overcome barriers of distance, workforce shortage, and stigma, but to be effective, they must be underpinned by rigorous science, cultural appropriateness, and policy support.

The COVID 19 pandemic, for all its tragedy, has created a unique moment in history to reimagine how we define and care for brain health. PCNS is the test case. If we succeed in addressing it through collaborative research, shared knowledge, and human centered care, we will not only help millions of people suffering today, but also set a new benchmark for future neurological care.

This chapter aims to provide a comprehensive overview of Post-COVID Neurological Syndrome. We examine its biological underpinnings, clinical features, diagnostic challenges, and implications for health systems. We highlight opportunities for innovation in care delivery, advocacy, and global collaboration, and most importantly, we issue a call to action to clinicians, researchers, educators, policymakers, and funders to recognize PCNS as a legitimate and urgent brain health priority.

As authors and clinicians, we bring both a scientific and personal commitment to this work. Since 2020, we have stood with our patients in clinics, hospitals, and community settings, witnessing the immense toll of this condition. We have also seen hope, courage, and recovery. This introduction, and the chapter that follows, is dedicated to those living with PCNS, and to those working to ensure their journey is met with understanding, care, and respect.

13.2 What We Tried to Say in This Book

This book was born out of necessity. Since the early days of the pandemic, we have witnessed something unusual. Patients who recovered from the initial viral illness continued to suffer. Their symptoms were vague but disabling. They could not think clearly. They could not return to work. They were exhausted. They had headaches, dizziness, numbness, anxiety, and depression. Many were dismissed or told it was in their head.

But we listened, and we took note. Slowly, a pattern emerged. What we were seeing was real. It had a name: Post-COVID Neurological Syndrome, PCNS.

This book is a response to that reality. It is a call to recognize PCNS as a serious and urgent global brain health challenge. It is our attempt to bring clarity, compassion, and coordination to a condition that has been misunderstood, misdiagnosed, and too often ignored.

Across the chapters, we have brought together voices from different parts of the world. We have examined the burden, the science, the stories, and the solutions. We have shown that PCNS is not rare. It is not mysterious. It is measurable. It is common, and it is deeply disruptive to daily life.

We began with a simple message. PCNS is real. It is disabling, and it is preventable and treatable—if we act together.

13.3 What Did We Cover?

We started with the global impact. PCNS is not limited to one country or one type of patient. It is present in high-income and low-income settings. It affects the young and the old. It affects healthcare workers, teachers, parents, children, and migrants. It affects people who had mild infections and those who were hospitalized.

We explored the data. The Global Burden of Disease framework now includes post-COVID conditions, yet the data still underestimate the problem. Why? Because PCNS is underdiagnosed, it is not well coded, and patients are falling through the cracks.

We unpacked the science. We discussed how PCNS is a brain-based disorder driven by chronic low grade inflammation. We talked about immune dysregulation, blood brain barrier breakdown, and neuropeptide dysfunction. These are not new ideas. They build on years of knowledge, but they have not yet been applied to PCNS with urgency.

We aligned our message with the World Health Organization's Intersectoral Global Action Plan. This plan calls for better neurological care, better data, better policy, and better inclusion of brain health in national agendas. PCNS is the perfect test case. If we succeed in addressing PCNS, we build a better system for all brain disorders.

We highlighted the barriers. There are so many: stigma, fragmented care, lack of funding, poor education, dismissive attitudes, silos in medicine and research. We mapped these obstacles and proposed ways to overcome them. We showed that these are not just medical barriers. They are social, economic, and political.

We made a case for services. We cannot wait for more evidence. We already have enough to act. We called for clinics, care pathways, and community supports that recognize PCNS as a legitimate health condition. We urged governments and health systems to act now, not later.

We focused on education. Too few doctors are trained in post-infectious syndromes. Too many patients are told their symptoms are stress. We need to educate medical students, general practitioners, specialists, and allied health workers. We need to build capacity, and we need to listen to patients as co educators.

We identified the research gaps. We do not yet know why some people develop PCNS and others do not. We need biomarkers. We need diagnostic tools. We need trials for new treatments. We need to study recovery, and we need to do all of this inclusively—with patients at the center.

We reviewed what treatment looks like today. It is patchy. Some patients are lucky. Most are not. Care is inconsistent. There are no guidelines. Some patients receive rehabilitation. Others receive nothing. We can do better. We must do better.

We also addressed patient needs. These are not just clinical. Patients need recognition. They need access. They need continuity. They need support, and they need to be heard. We need to reshape services around the lived experience.

We clarified the terminology. PCNS is different from long COVID. Long COVID is a broad umbrella. PCNS is a neurological syndrome, distinct, defined, and deserving of its own care model and research agenda.

We even explored PCNS in children. The effects are there: cognitive impairment, fatigue, learning disruption, mental health concerns. We cannot ignore this. The brain development of an entire generation may be at risk.

We shared a new approach: A systems neuroscience approach. Based on our work with functional testing and cognitive profiling, we outlined how a battery of simple tests could help diagnose and track PCNS. This opens the door to better triage, early intervention, and meaningful rehabilitation.

Finally, we concluded with a clear message. PCNS is not going away, but suffering is not inevitable. What we need is coordinated, multidisciplinary action from researchers, from clinicians, from governments, and from society.

13.4 PCNS, Brain Health, and SDG 3: A Shared Crisis, a Shared Opportunity

What is the price of being invisible?

We asked that question in our global advocacy work around headache disorders. Now we ask it again with Post-COVID Neurological Syndrome. Both conditions are silent burdens. Both disrupt the lives of millions. Both are misunderstood, and both are neglected—not just in medicine but in public health, education, economics, and social care.

PCNS is not just a medical issue. It is a development issue. It sits right at the intersection of the Sustainable Development Goals. Most importantly, it challenges our ability to deliver on *SDG 3: Good Health and Wellbeing for all at all ages.*

Let us be clear. PCNS is not rare. It is not marginal. It is not new, but like headache disorders, it has remained in the shadows. Not because the science is lacking, not because patients are few, but because we have not yet made brain health a global health priority.

We have the knowledge. We have the tools. What we need is courage, coordination, and commitment.

13.5 What Does PCNS Share with Headache Disorders?

First, both are *highly disabling*. Headache disorders are the second most disabling condition globally. PCNS has rapidly joined the ranks of leading causes of disability, especially among working-age people and women. The symptoms may look different, but the impact is the same: lost productivity, social isolation, mental health burden, missed opportunities, years lost to poor quality of life.

Second, both are *poorly funded*. Compared to conditions like cancer or heart disease, headache and PCNS receive a fraction of the research investment. Funding for post-viral syndromes remains scattered. Most national funding agencies still do not have dedicated streams for PCNS. Global neurological research spending is under 2% of total health research funding.

Third, both suffer from *stigma and disbelief*. Patients are too often told "it's just stress." They are passed from one specialist to another. They face long delays in diagnosis. They are told their symptoms are imaginary, or worse, their fault. This is particularly true for women, culturally and linguistically diverse communities, and people with disabilities.

Fourth, both lack *structured care pathways*. Most health systems have no dedicated clinics, guidelines, or referral systems for PCNS. Services for headache are just as patchy. This leaves patients navigating a maze. Many fall through the cracks. Others give up, and those who persist are left managing complex conditions with little coordinated support.

Fifth, both are *treatable and manageable*. This is the real tragedy. We have evidence based strategies to help these patients: lifestyle interventions, psychological therapies, physical rehabilitation, medications, peer support, education, digital tools. These are not futuristic solutions. They are available now, but they are not deployed widely, or equitably, or early enough.

13.6 Where Does SDG 3 Come In?

SDG 3 is the promise the world made to improve health and wellbeing for all. It is not just about survival. It is about thriving. It is about access. It is about leaving no one behind.

PCNS tests that promise.

It reveals the fault lines in our systems. It exposes who is valued, who is believed, who gets care. It reminds us that recovery is not just a medical task—it is a societal one, and it proves that unless we include brain health in our health development agenda, SDG 3 cannot be achieved.

PCNS fits under almost every SDG 3 target:

- 3.4: Reduce premature mortality from non-communicable diseases and promote mental health and wellbeing
- 3.8: Achieve universal health coverage, including financial risk protection and access to essential services
- 3.c: Substantially increase health financing and the recruitment, development, and training of the health workforce
- 3.d: Strengthen the capacity of all countries for early warning, risk reduction, and management of health risks

But SDG 3 is not just about healthcare. It is about fairness, equity, and systems. PCNS intersects with *SDG 4 (education)*, *SDG 5 (gender equality)*, *SDG 8 (decent work)*, and *SDG 10 (reducing inequalities)*.

When a child with PCNS cannot concentrate at school, that is an education issue.
When a working mother with PCNS cannot get time off, that is a workplace policy issue.
When an older migrant struggles to access post-COVID care in their language, that is a justice issue.
When a patient in a rural area cannot get to a clinic, that is a systems design issue.

The promise of SDG 3 is only real if it includes people with PCNS.

13.7 The Power of Framing PCNS as a Development Issue

Framing PCNS as a development challenge changes the conversation. It moves us beyond narrow biomedical models. It opens the door to multisectoral action. It brings new stakeholders to the table. It allows us to speak to ministries of education, employment, housing, digital infrastructure. It makes space for community, culture, and care.

We have seen how this works with headache advocacy. When we connected migraine to lost productivity, school dropouts, and suicide prevention, governments began to listen. We can do the same for PCNS.

PCNS is not just a viral aftermath. It is a test of health system resilience. It is a signal of inequality. It is a model for integrated care. It is a proving ground for preventive brain health.

13.8 What Would Success Look Like?

Success would mean PCNS is:

- Officially recognized in health policy frameworks

- Included in ICD classifications and burden of disease models
- Addressed in clinical training programs across all health professions
- Funded as a priority research area
- Cared for in interdisciplinary clinics with community partnerships
- Supported by digital and remote care platforms
- Spoken about in public health campaigns without stigma
- Included in national brain health strategies
- Measured, evaluated, and monitored through better data

Success would mean patients are not alone.
Clinicians are not guessing.
Researchers are not scrambling for support.
Policymakers are not ignoring the evidence.

It would mean we are truly walking the talk of SDG 3.

13.9 We Know What to Do

Throughout this book, we have laid out a path forward.

We need to break the silos.
We need to fund translational research.
We need to build care pathways that start at the community level.
We need to embed lived experience into design, delivery, and review.
We need to train a new generation of clinicians who understand systems, not just symptoms.
We need digital tools that enhance—not replace—compassionate care.
We need governments to put brain health on the map.

And we need global partnerships: WHO, WFN, WFNR, Academic networks, Patient organizations, Industry. They all have a role.

We are not starting from scratch.
We are not working in the dark.
What we need is political will.

And the belief that these patients matter.

13.10 A Shared Message Across All Chapters

In every chapter of this book, we have told a part of this story.

From epidemiology to systems neuroscience.

From pediatric care to patient lived experience.
From low income countries to major academic centers.
From definitions to diagnostics to service delivery.

We have shown that PCNS is a legitimate, life altering neurological condition that deserves attention.

We have also shown that with the right tools, the right framing, and the right partnerships, PCNS can be addressed, not in ten years, but now.

13.11 Conclusion

This is not just a book about a post-viral condition.

It is a book about change.
It is a book about connection.
It is a book about doing things better—for the brain, for the body, and for the whole person.

By linking PCNS to the broader movement for brain health and SDG 3, we can elevate it. We can fund it. We can care for it properly.

And in doing so, we may finally answer that question we started with:

What is the price of being invisible?
Too high.
Much too high.

Now is the time to see, to act, and to deliver.

13.12 What Do We Hope to Achieve?

We want to shift the narrative. PCNS is not imaginary. It is not psychological. It is not a mystery. It is a brain-based syndrome. We want to normalize discussion of PCNS. We want to make it visible.

We want PCNS to be recognized in global disease classification systems. We want national health systems to establish dedicated PCNS clinics. We want more funding for PCNS research. We want health professionals to be trained to diagnose and manage PCNS. We want digital health and mobile tools to be deployed to support patients.

We want equity. PCNS does not affect all communities equally: women, people from culturally and linguistically diverse backgrounds, people living in poverty, and people with disability face the highest burden. We must design policies that are inclusive and fair.

We want collaboration. PCNS is not a challenge for one field. It is a challenge for everyone: neurology, immunology, rehabilitation, psychiatry, public health, general practice, nursing, policy, lived experience. We must work together.

And we want hope. Many people recover from PCNS, but recovery takes time. It takes support. It takes belief. We want this book to be a signal of hope to every patient who has been dismissed or doubted. We see you. We believe you. We are working for you.

13.13 In Closing

This book is not the end of the story. It is the beginning of a global conversation. It is a blueprint. It is an invitation.

To clinicians: open your eyes and ears to PCNS. Believe your patients. Learn from them. Work with them.

To researchers: ask better questions. Break the silos. Share your data.

To educators: teach the next generation to care for patients with complex post-infectious syndromes.

To policymakers: fund the clinics, the trials, the registries, and the services we so urgently need.

To patients and carers: your voice matters. Keep speaking. Keep fighting. Keep hoping.

Let us move from scattered efforts to united action, from delay to delivery, from suffering to recovery.

Let this be the decade we got PCNS right.

Further Reading

Aamodt AH, Stovner LJ, Hagen K, Zwart JA. Comorbidity of headache and psychiatric disorders in the general population: the HUNT study. J Headache Pain. 2006;7(4):210–9.

Collaborators, G.B.D. 2019 Diseases and Injuries. Global burden of 369 diseases and injuries in 204 countries and territories, 1990–2019: a systematic analysis. Lancet. 2020;396(10258):1204–22.

Crewther S, Wijeratne T. Post-COVID Neurological Syndrome: conceptual framework and systems-based understanding. Brain Behav Immun Health. 2021;17:100339.

Davis HE, Assaf GS, McCorkell L, Wei H, Low RJ, Re'em Y, Redfield S, Austin JP, Akrami A, The Patient-Led Research Collaborative. Characterizing long COVID in an international cohort: 7 months of symptoms and their impact. EClinicalMedicine. 2021;38:101019.

Fukuda K, Straus SE, Hickie I, Sharpe MC, Dobbins JG, Komaroff A. The chronic fatigue syndrome: a comprehensive approach to its definition and study. Ann Intern Med. 1994;121(12):953–9.

GBD 2021 COVID-19 Collaborators. Global burden of COVID-19 restrictions and post-acute consequences: a systematic review and meta-analysis. Lancet Public Health. 2022;7(10):e828–37.

Graham EL, Clark JR, Orban ZS, Lim PH, Szymanski AL, Taylor C, DiBiase RM, Jia DT, Balabanov R, Ho SU, Batra A. Persistent neurologic symptoms and cognitive dysfunction in non-hospitalized COVID-19 long haulers. Ann Clin Transl Neurol. 2021;8(5):1073–85.

Institute for Health Metrics and Evaluation (IHME). Global Burden of Disease Study 2021 (GBD 2021). *Seattle*: *IHME*; 2022. Available at: https://www.healthdata.org/gbd.

Nasserie T, Hittle M, Goodman SN. Assessment of the frequency and variety of persistent symptoms among patients with COVID-19: a systematic review. JAMA Netw Open. 2021;4(5):e2111417.

Rajan S, Khunti K, Alwan N, Steves C, Greenhalgh T, MacDermott N, Rammelt C, The WHO European Office for Long COVID. Policy brief: long COVID – preparing for the long haul. World Health Organization Europe; 2021.

Stovner LJ, Nichols E, Steiner TJ, Abd-Allah F, Abdelalim A, Al-Raddadi RM, Ansha MG, Barac A, Bekele BB, Fereshtehnejad SM, GBD 2016 Headache Collaborators. Global, regional, and national burden of migraine and tension-type headache, 1990–2016: a systematic analysis for the Global Burden of Disease Study 2016. Lancet Neurol. 2018;17(11):954–76.

Taquet M, Geddes JR, Husain M, Luciano S, Harrison PJ. 6-month neurological and psychiatric outcomes in 236 379 survivors of COVID-19: a retrospective cohort study using electronic health records. Lancet Psychiatry. 2021;8(5):416–27.

United Nations. Transforming our world: the 2030 Agenda for Sustainable Development. United Nations; 2015. Available at: https://sdgs.un.org/2030agenda.

WHO. Headache Disorders and Public Health: Education and Management Implications. World Health Organization. 2016. Available at: https://www.who.int/publications/i/item/9789241569534.

Wijeratne T, Crewther SG. Post-COVID 19 Neurological Syndrome (PCNS); a novel syndrome with challenges for the global neurology community. J Neurol Sci. 2020;419:117179.

World Health Organization. Intersectoral global action plan on epilepsy and other neurological disorders 2022–2031. Geneva: WHO; 2022. Available at: https://www.who.int/publications/i/item/9789240054567.

MIX
Papier aus verantwortungsvollen Quellen
Paper from responsible sources
FSC® C105338

If you have any concerns about our products,
you can contact us on
ProductSafety@springernature.com

In case Publisher is established outside the EU,
the EU authorized representative is:
Springer Nature Customer Service Center GmbH
Europaplatz 3, 69115 Heidelberg, Germany

Printed by Libri Plureos GmbH
in Hamburg, Germany